The
Naturopathic Way

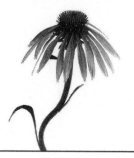

The
Naturopathic
Way

How to Detox, Find Quality Nutrition, and Restore Your Acid-Alkaline Balance

Christopher Vasey, N.D.

Translated by Jon E. Graham

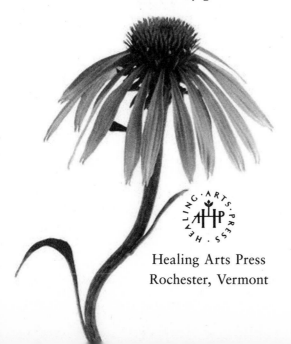

Healing Arts Press
Rochester, Vermont

Healing Arts Press
One Park Street
Rochester, Vermont 05767
www.HealingArtsPress.com

Healing Arts Press is a division of Inner Traditions International

Originally published in French under the title *Petit traité de naturopathie à l'usage des malades qui veulent retrouver la santé et des bien-portants qui veulent le rester: suivi du Dictionnaire thématique des concepts de la naturopathie* by Éditions Jouvence, S.A., Chemin du Guillon 20, Case 143, CH-1233 Genève-Bernex, Switzerland, www.editions-jouvence.com, info@editions-jouvence.com

Note to the reader: This book is intended as an informational guide. The remedies, approaches, and techniques described herein are meant to supplement, and not to be a substitute for, professional medical care or treatment. They should not be used to treat a serious ailment without prior consultation with a qualified health care professional.

Library of Congress Cataloging-in-Publication Data

Vasey, Christopher.
   [Petit traité de naturopathie. English.]
   The naturopathic way : how to detox, find quality nutrition, and restore your acid-alkaline balance / Christopher Vasey ; translated by Jon E. Graham.
      p. cm.
   Originally published in French under the title: Petit traité de naturopathie: à l'usage des malades qui veulent retrouver la santé et des bien-portants qui veulent le rester: suivi du Dictionnaire thématique des concepts de la naturopathie. Genève : Éditions Jouvence, c2007.
   Includes bibliographical references and index.
   Summary: "How naturopathy works to establish good health and protect against the toxic causes of illness."—Provided by publisher.
   ISBN 978-1-59477-260-3 (pbk.)
   1. Naturopathy. I. Title.
   RZ440.V3713 2007
   615.5'35—dc22
                                                                              2008041957

Printed and bound in the United States by Lake Book Manufacturing

10   9   8   7   6   5   4   3   2   1

Text design and layout by Virginia Scott Bowman
This book was typeset in Sabon with New Baskerville and Avenir as display typefaces

Contents

ॐ

Foreword

꙳

Our medical system is ill, and Western society, like the rest of our planet, is not faring well. Iatrogenic illnesses (illnesses actually caused by allopathic treatments) and nosocomial illnesses (those that develop in hospitals) are increasing at an alarming rate. We promise the children being born today that they will live to see one hundred, but we are confusing medicated old age with an enjoyable quality of life.

At the same time, it's been demonstrated that 90 percent of all cancers are linked to nutritional and environmental factors. Doctors are developing more and more cases of depression in the two years following establishment of their professional practices.

Should our response to these paradoxes of the modern world be to maintain our comfort level with an ostrichlike denial of the evidence, or to hold an alarmist and paranoid discourse? Naturopathy believes that this picture, dramatic as it may be, can be studied calmly and solved positively if we can manage to awaken the awareness of both consumers and decision makers, most of whose views have been framed by a single philosophy.

In fact, whether it involves ecoplanetary or health

imbalances, everything rests on the philosophy, points of reference, and points of view that determine human behavior. Most of the problems we currently face have their origin in materialistic thinking and the egotistical belief that humanity can operate independently of the laws of nature or biology.

Naturopathy's chosen objective is health and well-being, but in the framework of a profound and authentic reconciliation with these laws, which are often simple and full of common sense: How do we best nourish ourselves, breathe freely, and take care of our bodies and their natural elimination processes? How do we optimize our sleep, our vitality, and our libido? How do we recharge ourselves through the natural elements—earth, water, air, and light, for example? Why should we carefully alternate times of activity and times of rest? How can we purify and regenerate the internal cellular environment of our bodies? How can we be consumers without endangering our planetary resources?

Good sense such as this is to be found, in fact, where it has always been: in the heart of the great health-sustaining recommendations and medical traditions that date back to the fabled teachings of the Sumerians and the Essenes. This includes Ayurvedic, Native American, Chinese, and Tibetan practices, and more specifically for us in the Western world, Hippocrates' noble philosophy. The most surprising thing, perhaps, is that beyond the contextual differences in their details, all of these traditions are based on the same foundations, and only allopathic medicine (the institutional Western form that prevails in most of the world today) has been established in total opposition to these universal concepts.

What, then, are the common elements in these traditions? Prevention is preferable to healing, teaching is preferable to treating, and giving the individual responsibility for his or her health is preferable to taking charge. Other common features include considering the whole person rather than the symptom, remaining humbly and respectfully attuned to the laws of a healthy life, and working with the energetic processes of regeneration and spontaneous self-healing rather than putting your faith in the effectiveness of a remedy. In short, an entire program.

After more than a century in the United States and seventy years in Europe, naturopathy has become the discipline that offers another kind of medicine, one in which the practitioner is first and foremost an educator of health, perfectly effective in the treatment of all the chronic diseases—the so-called functional diseases—as well as in primary prevention and quality of life. This does not make the naturopath just one more practitioner in the vast field of natural medicine that includes, for example, phytotherapy and homeopathy. He remains, rather, the general practitioner of health, as the allopathic physician is the general practitioner of illness. Is it now possible to envision the ideal public health system—perhaps modeled after the integrated medicine practiced in some parts of the United States—in which the allopathic doctor, the natural medicine practitioner, and the naturopath can congenially complement one another's services in an atmosphere of perfect mutual respect, all for the benefit of the patient?

The French Federation of Naturopathy (FENAHMAN) states that naturopathy is founded on the principle of the vital energy of the body, and that it combines the practices that have emerged from Western tradition based on the ten natural aspects of health: diet, hydration, psychology, physical exercise, respiration, plants, reflexology, light therapy, and manual and energetic techniques. It aims at preserving and optimizing the overall health and quality of life of an individual by allowing the body to regenerate itself through natural means. Faithful to these concepts, my colleague Christopher Vasey has realized a work of remarkable synthesis here, because it is no easy task to summarize the essence of our art, as well as its useful application, in so few pages. He's earned my great respect for his precision, and my sincerest congratulations for his teaching ability.

In this work, we have the pleasure of rediscovering the essential keys of the five columns treasured by Hippocrates and all of our European teachers (Sebastian Kneipp, Paul Carton, Henri Durville, Pierre Valentin Marchesseau, André Roux), and North American teachers (Benedict Lust, John H. Tilden, Henry Lindlahr, Bernarr Macfadden, Bernard Jensen), namely: serology, the science of bodily fluids and their disorders (excesses, deficiencies, obstructions); vitalism, the study of our intrinsic vital energy and its invaluable capabilities (homeostasis, regeneration, self-healing); prevention, maintaining our connection with the natural world and a wholesome lifestyle; causalism, the methodical quest for the primary origin of symptoms, which always comes back to not only the condition of the bodily fluids, but also the energetic state, meaning psychology, spirituality, or ecology; and holism, the global approach to the human being and the way he interacts with his environment.

Thank you, Christopher, for this new reference work, and pleasant reading to all.

DANIEL KIEFFER

Daniel Kieffer is the president of FENAHMAN, which is the French Federation of Naturopathy, and president of the UEN, the European Union of Naturopathy. He is also the director of CENATHO, the European College of Traditional Holistic Naturopathy, and a member of OMNES, which is the Organization of Natural Medicine and Health Education.

Introduction

❦

For many people, naturopathy distinguishes itself from allopathic medicine only by the remedies it employs. These remedies are natural (found in nature—medicinal plants, hydrotherapy, and so forth) rather than "chemical" (created in a laboratory). In reality there is another stark difference: the naturopath has a completely different concept of disease from that of the allopathic physician.

Naturopathy, therefore, does not do the same thing by different means, but actually does something quite different, using extremely dissimilar means. Its therapeutic objectives are, in fact, governed by a completely different logic.

What is this logic?

The purpose of this book is to present the different aspects of naturopathy by revealing the foundations on which it is based (theoretical framework), and by describing the means it uses to bring relief to the sufferers of illness (practical application).

1

The Naturopathic Concept of Illness

ॐ

WHAT IS AN ILLNESS?

*The Importance of the Body's Internal
Cellular Environment*

It is rare for any person whose health has been compromised to ask himself, "Why am I sick? What is really happening in my body?" To the contrary, all of his attention—and that of those around him—is focused on his blatant, disagreeable, or painful symptoms, which are actually just surface manifestations of his deep-rooted illness.

It seems self-evident that the normal reaction would be to make a vigorous counterattack to the assault represented by the illness. As a general rule we behave as if disease were an outside entity independent of the patient, which, by entering the body, suddenly makes the patient sick. From this perspective, we consider the individual stricken by illness to be an innocent victim requiring our assistance because, through bad luck, he or she suffered an unhealthy assault.

The expressions used to speak of illness clearly support this premise. We say that we "fall" ill, that we have been "stricken," or that we have "caught" a disease.

According to this hypothesis, taught by allopathic medicine, each "assailant" determines different characteristic disorders. There are, therefore, as many diseases as there are assailants; this is what is known as multiple causes, or the plurality of disease. Since there are no common elements among diseases in this framework, each must be treated with its own specific remedy.

What Is Allopathic Medicine?

Allopathic medicine is a therapeutic method that deals with disease by using methods that, generally speaking, oppose the curative effects of the body's vital forces. By suppressing toxins into the depths of the body, antisymptom remedies do banish the symptoms from the surface, but this is to the detriment of the biological terrain.

In naturopathy, however, all diseases are considered as different manifestations of a single, common disorder. This common denominator, this profound illness from which all others result, resides on the level of the biological terrain, or internal cellular environment. This terrain consists of all the fluids in the body, including those contained within cells and those in which the cells are bathed, as well as the blood, lymph, and cerebrospinal fluid.

How Is Naturopathy Different from Allopathy?

Naturopathy treats disease using natural methods, and takes action to improve the biological terrain rather than to diminish the symptoms. In supporting the body's own healing power, it addresses the deep roots of illness, rather than the effects.

The intra- and extracellular fluids, along with the blood, represent 70 percent of the body's weight. These fluids are crucial, inasmuch as they constitute the environment of our cells. Intracellular fluid fills the cells, gives the body its shape and tone, and allows the exchanges that need to take place between the organs. Extracellular fluid carries oxygen and nutrients to the cells, and carries waste from the cells to the excretory organs.

Our cells depend entirely on these fluids. They deliver nutritive supplies (food, vitamins, water, oxygen, and so

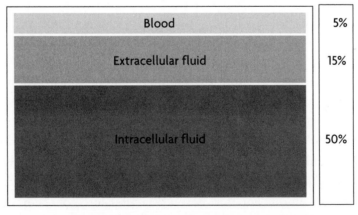

The bodily fluids that make up the internal cellular environment and their weight percentages in the body

on), eliminate toxins created by the metabolic process, and transmit messages from one cell to another, ensuring their coordinated and harmonious interaction.

Just as our environment provides conditions that are favorable for health or that make us sick, depending on whether or not it is polluted, the environment of the cells plays an influential role in the state of their health. If they are bathing in a milieu that is deficient in oxygen and overloaded with wastes, they will be incapable of performing their tasks properly.

Health: A Definition

Health is not the absence of detectable disease symptoms, but corresponds to a state of the biological terrain in which the composition of the bodily fluids ensures and provides the conditions favorable to the cells' unhampered normal activity. Health is determined by the state of the body's internal cellular environment. If this biological terrain is healthy, then the body is healthy; if it is unhealthy, the body is ill, even if there are no apparent symptoms.

Our body is made up of cells. If these cells are not functioning normally, the entire body will function poorly and enter the state that we call illness.

There is a precise and ideal composition of the internal environment that permits proper functioning of the body. Any major quantitative or qualitative change in these fluids leads to illness. For this reason, the vital force of the body is constantly struggling to maintain the internal cellular environment in perfect balance.

The body does this primarily by neutralizing and expelling all wastes and toxins that are a consequence of metabolism. This purification is carried out by the emunctory, or excretory organs—liver, intestines, kidneys, skin, lungs—which filter and eliminate waste.

Health, therefore, is founded on a very precarious state of balance that must be constantly restored. For example, if the body's biological terrain becomes overloaded on an irregular basis with small amounts of toxins—caused by overeating, or ingesting a stimulant like alcohol, or certain medications—the consequences won't be dramatic because the body is perfectly capable of purifying itself and restoring the ideal composition of bodily fluids. On the other hand, if these unhealthy incidents start becoming regular or daily habits, the body's capacity for restoring its own balance will be quickly exceeded.

These wastes accumulate in the bloodstream, which eventually deposits them along the walls of the blood vessels. As the diameter of the blood vessels shrinks and the blood itself becomes thicker, blood circulation becomes less and less effective. The exchanges made between the blood and the cellular fluids slow down. The wastes that cells are constantly discharging collect in the tissue instead of being flushed rapidly out of the body. The organs of the body, increasingly saturated with wastes, are unable to perform their work properly, and the congested excretory organs are no longer able to guarantee sufficient purification of the bodily fluids. All of the body's activities are then thrown out of kilter, whether these activities involve the cells, the enzymes, white blood cells, or biochemical reactions.

This constricted state of the body's internal cellular environment is what natural medicine considers to be the intrinsic illness.

This state can be found in all diseases. It forms both their unique characteristics and their common base. So it is not because an illness "enters" the body that its overall state deteriorates; it is because the state of the biological terrain has been degraded that illness manifests.

Since bodily fluids never stop circulating and there are constant exchanges taking place among them, toxins will necessarily spread throughout the body, and not a single part of the body will be spared. Hence this fundamental aphorism of natural medicine: "Illness has one cause—it is the congested state of the biological terrain." This concept of one unique malady, the unity of disease—that all health disorders are the expression of a single illness, which is the degradation of the biological terrain—is the opposite of the premise of multiple causes for diseases that is found in standard (allopathic) medicine.

At first glance there would seem to be a contradiction between this concept of the unique illness and clearly differentiated forms of disease with which we are familiar. Naturopathy, however, considers every local disorder not as an illness in its own right, but as merely the surface manifestation of a deeper problem, a result of preexisting obstruction. This illness could not make its presence known unless the internal cellular environment had already been overloaded with wastes. The specific local disorder it causes is comparable to the tip of the iceberg. The biggest part of the iceberg remains invisible: it is the overloaded biological terrain.

Local disorders are, therefore, not intrinsic illnesses but simply the secondary consequences of the root malady: the biological terrain overloaded with wastes. Hence another aphorism of natural medicine, "There are no local diseases; there are only general diseases."

This is clearly the case because local disorders evolve as a result of the state of the biological terrain: the more it deteriorates, the more the disorder escalates. Whether the local disorder is a case of the flu or a cancerous tumor, the process is the same. The increase in the rate of the body's overload—toxins that dangerously burden the biological terrain when they collect in overly large quantities—aggravates the illness and encourages the development of the disorder. Conversely, the local symptoms will diminish proportionately with a reduction in the rate of toxic overload. They will vanish entirely when the terrain has recovered its stasis, in situations when this return to a balanced state is still possible.

The localization of "surface" disorders depends on the particular weaknesses of an individual's body. All the body's organs are immersed in fluids that are overloaded with wastes. They are all irritated and attacked similarly by toxic sludge. The first organs to give way, the first to find this environment intolerable, are obviously those that are genetically weakest or have the greatest demands placed on them. For example, for people whose profession requires them to talk a lot, it would be the throat; for those most often affected by stress, the nerves will give way; miners, painters, and others who breathe in dust or noxious gases at their place of employment are likely to have problems with the respiratory tract. The illness is one and the same in all cases, but manifests differently in every individual.

We owe this concept of a single cause for every disease to Hippocrates, known as the father of medicine. In the time around 500 BCE he wrote: "The nature of all illness is the same. It differs only in its seat. I think it only reveals itself in such diversity because of the multiplicity of places where the illness is established. In fact, its essence is one, and the cause producing it is also one."

Twenty-five centuries later, Alexis Carrel, the 1912 Nobel Prize winner for medicine, stated: "The body is ill in its entirety. No illness remains strictly confined to a single organ."

> ༀ
>
> When the state of the biological terrain deteriorates, illness appears. Every local disorder is only the surface manifestation of a deeper disorder: the congestion of the body's internal cellular environment.

WHY DO WE FALL ILL?

The Role Played by Toxins and Deficiencies

When we understand how the state of the terrain becomes degraded, we also realize that it depends entirely on outside sustenance to build and renew itself. The nutritive substances contained in the foods we eat are used to manufacture cells and bodily fluids. Our bodies function thanks to them.

If the intake supplied by one's diet is greater than the body's needs, the body accumulates substances it is unable to use. As the body is forced to store them, they collect in the tissues. This can include chemical or synthetic ingredients in food, such as coloring, preservatives, and so on. Since nature has never provided any instructions to the body for their use, these more or less toxic substances will collect in the tissues and alter the biological terrain in accordance with their specific characteristics.

Even when the diet—the body's primary source for retaining or restoring health—is adequate, it is still possible for wastes to accumulate in the body. This occurs every time that worry, stress, fear, and so forth disturb the multitude of biochemical transformations that take place in the body—the body's metabolism. Digestion functions poorly, so the foods ingested engender a plethora of wastes, generally designated as toxins. This includes crystals, which, produced by the metabolism of proteins, are acidic in nature and can be hard and painful to excrete; and colloidal wastes, such as phlegm, which are produced by the metabolism of starches and fats and do not generally cause pain.

THE TWO KINDS OF TOXINS

	Crystals	Colloidal Wastes
Sources	proteins, white sugar, acidifying foods	starches, fats
Excretory organs responsible for elimination	kidneys, sweat glands	liver, gallbladder, intestines, sebaceous glands, lungs

All of these substances, whether toxic or not, when present in excess amounts prevent the body from functioning properly and are considered to be the primary cause of the deterioration of the biological terrain, and therefore the source of disease.

The body may also become overloaded with wastes due to the poor breakdown and utilization of food substances caused by a lack of physical activity and the insufficient oxygenation that results from a sedentary lifestyle. Additionally, when the excretory organs designed for the elimination of toxins are not working efficiently, the body is compelled to store the retained wastes in its tissues.

Normal cellular activity also produces wastes, but only a fairly minimal amount. There is a much greater danger when the cells are diseased. They then can release far greater amounts of wastes that gradually will poison the entire body.

The factors that come into play with regard to the deterioration and congestion of the biological terrain are, therefore, multiple, but in all cases involve wastes formed by poorly metabolized ingested substances. This is why life hygiene, meaning personal health care, and vigilance about nutritious foods are so vitally important.

The food, beverages, medication, and stimulants that we consume can either keep our biological terrain healthy and disease resistant, or cause it to deteriorate.

∾∾

There is another major cause for degradation of the biological terrain, one brought about not by an excess of one or more substances in the body, but by a deficiency in a substance it requires to function properly.

A deficiency is a lack of essential nutrients that are indispensable for the body's ability to rebuild itself and function. Such nutrients include proteins, carbohydrates, fats, minerals, vitamins, and trace elements. The composition of the body's internal environment can be maintained only when there is sufficient intake of all the elements it requires. If one of these elements is not supplied in sufficient quantity, there is an immediate slowdown in physical function. When this element is entirely lacking from the diet, the body functions that are dependent on it can no longer be assured. If this state of complete deficiency extends for a prolonged amount of time, death is a real possibility.

In our society of abundance, it might seem difficult to imagine falling ill due to dietary deficiencies, but the truth is it is very possible and even quite easy. The foods available today supply less and less of our body's needs because they themselves are suffering deficiencies, due to modern farming and husbandry practices. The countless refining processes our food undergoes before reaching the grocery shelves exacerbates the problem.

Another cause of deficiency resides not in the inadequate intake of nutrients, but in their destruction by chemical ingredients in foods and medications, substances that act as anti-vitamins or inhibit the activity of trace elements. Specialized diets, those which systematically exclude certain kinds of food (for example, carbohydrates), also contribute to the production of deficiencies because of the lack of variety in the foods they provide the body.

When deficiencies are present for an extended time—which is the case when poor eating habits are maintained—they create substantial changes in the composition of bodily fluids and cause an insidious, gradual weakening of the body's resistance.

Furthermore, because most nutritive elements work interdependently to ensure their most effective use by the body, a deficiency in any one of them will create a series of other deficiencies, in a chain reaction.

A body suffering from nutrient deficiencies functions less well and eliminates waste poorly. Consequently, the ratio of excess waste and toxin in the body will only increase.

THE TWO CAUSES OF DETERIORATION OF THE BIOLOGICAL TERRAIN

Overloads	Deficiencies
Toxins (urea, uric acid); toxin-creating substances (tobacco, alcohol, coffee); food additives (food coloring, preservatives); poisons from pollution (lead, cadmium)	Water, oxygen, proteins, carbohydrates, fats, vitamins, minerals, trace elements

Illness arises, therefore, when the biological terrain is overloaded with wastes and is suffering from deficiencies. The functioning of the body is disrupted and can no longer defend itself properly. This phenomenon is not as unknown as it may appear, as it is used strategically in standard medical research. In fact, for studying bacterial activity or testing new remedies, animals are inoculated with germs. If these animals are enjoying good health, and their internal cellular environments are experiencing neither overloads nor deficiencies, infections either do not appear, or do so with much less frequency.

The way modern medical science attempts to overcome this obstacle to experimentation speaks volumes: healthy animals are made susceptible to bacterial attack through a "scientific" devastation of their biological terrain. They are fed deficient food that is not adapted to their digestive capabilities, too much food, cooked food, and chemical cocktails. A stress condition is created in the animals by placing them in darkness, putting their feet in cold water, and so forth.

༄

Disease arises when the body is overloaded with waste and is suffering deficiencies.

HOW DO WE HEAL?

The Wisdom of the Body

Everyone has, at least once, recovered from a disease without taking any medicine, or products containing active ingredients for treating illness. And yet, when someone is sick, the main concern is always to procure medication. This need for a remedy at any cost has been engraved deeply into our brains, as it is commonly accepted that without medicine there is no recovery.

Medications are supposed to contain all the curative powers necessary to restore a sick body to health. And yet, how many patients have recovered their health without taking any medication, either because it was unavailable or because they simply did not want to take medication? Also, how do animals cure themselves, since they do not have any medicines naturally available to them? Is there another option?

Natural medicine talks about a "medicalizing" nature or "vital force of the body." This force cannot be identified with any one organ of the body; its existence is revealed only in the effects of its action. Hippocrates said, "The vital force of the body is the most powerful force of cohesion and action in existence. However, it is invisible to the eye; only reasoning can conceive of it."

Vital Force

The vital force organizes living matter and orchestrates, synchronizes, and harmonizes all its organic functions. It is intangible and therefore cannot be identified with any single organ of the body. Its existence is revealed only by its effects. All its efforts are aimed at maintaining the body in an optimum state of health. It is this force that enlivens the organs and governs the processes of respiration, circulation, digestion, exchanges, and elimination. It also triggers reactions by the body's defense system; it scars wounds, neutralizes poisons, and prompts healing crises.

In the healthy state, the vital force orchestrates and harmonizes all physical functions of the body. It works constantly to maintain the body in the healthiest state possible.

In the event of injury, it is the vital force that directs the repair of tissue by scarring over wounds. When the body is attacked by products that threaten its integrity, whether they originate on the outside (venom, poison, microbes, and so on) or inside (toxins and metabolic waste), it puts the entire body on alert and implements its defense system.

When confronted by a rising tide of overloads and congestion of the tissues, the vital force does not remain on the sidelines as a passive spectator. It reacts vigorously to restore order to the physical organism so that it can continue—or resume—its normal functioning. All its efforts aim at reestablishing the purity of the biological terrain by neutralizing the toxins found in this internal cellular environment, and expelling waste from the body by means of the various excretory organs. This eviction of toxins from the body often can take a spectacular form. Such events are called detoxification crises, also known as cleansing crises, or healing crises, due to the abrupt intensity of their inception.

Elimination during these kinds of crises will be made through the same excretory organs as in conditions of normal health, but with greater forcefulness. Colloidal waste will be expectorated through the respiratory tract, and urine will be laden with waste. The skin may eliminate waste through heavy perspiration, pimples, or various forms of eczema. The digestive tract also plays a role by releasing diarrhea, or abundant secretions of bile.

Which excretory organs are pressed into service depends on the nature of the waste and the strength of a patient's different organs, so there are significant variations from one individual to the next, and multiple possibilities for the localization of disorders. These local disorders are the visible manifestation of the vital force's defensive reaction as it seeks to correct a much more profound ill: the congestion of the biological terrain.

In standard medicine, every local defensive reaction is catalogued according to its characteristics, is given a specific name, and is then considered an illness in its own right. The eliminatory nature of illness is something Hippocrates proclaimed centuries ago: "All diseases are resolved either by the mouth, the bowels, the bladder, or some other such organ. Sweat is a common form of resolution in all these cases." The seventeenth-century English physician Thomas Sydenham wrote: "A disease, however much its cause may be adverse to the human body, is nothing more than an effort of nature, who strives with might and main to restore the health of the patient by the elimination of the morbific [disease-causing] humor." Closer to our time, in 1924, Dr. Paul Carton—the Hippocrates of the twentieth century—stated: "Disease in reality is only the translation of an inner effort to neutralize and clean out toxins, which the body performs for preservation and regeneration and is not an effort to destroy health . . . "

The body is, therefore, quite capable of working all alone toward its own healing. Thanks to the vital force, it contains the capacity for self-healing through its immune response. Hippocrates called this ability of the vital force its "medicalizing" nature.

The immune response is the body's capacity to resist and defend itself when confronted with disease-causing processes. It is present in the body from birth, and remains present in both sickness and in health. But the body's immune system is only powerful and effective as long as the biological terrain remains pure and balanced. Looking at it from the reverse perspective, the more the biological terrain is saturated with waste and deficient in other substances it requires for health, the greater the reduction in the body's ability to defend itself.

The different elements of the immune system (bone marrow, lymph nodes, white blood cells, and so forth) are also bathing in the bodily fluids, and their effectiveness is dependent on the quality of these fluids. The degradation of the biological terrain can become so pronounced—either because the toxic overload is so great, the deficit of nutrients so profound, or both, as is most often the case—that the immune system loses, for all practical purposes, its ability to take action. The body is then left almost defenseless against assaults.

Although natural medicine considers the internal cellular environment of the body to be the deciding factor in health, the harmful influence of germs is not minimized. Germs, viruses, and parasites are a reality and represent a certain potential danger to the human body. It would be inaccurate, however, to consider them to be the primary cause of disease. A good many illnesses are not due to a bacterial attack. For example, heart failure, diabetes, asthma, digestive disorders, and nervous disorders are not caused by germs. Furthermore, the immune system, if it is functioning properly, is capable of defending the body against all microbial attacks. If this were not the case, the human race would have vanished from the face of the earth long ago.

There is a subtle balance between the body's defensive force and its vulnerability to attacks from germs. The stronger the immune system is, the sooner germs are rendered powerless or destroyed. They can enter the body but not cause any damage. On the other hand, the weaker the body's defense system, the more germs can develop, proliferate, and invade the entire body with their devastating activity. The now-famous phrase attributed to Pasteur on his deathbed sums it up admirably: "The germ is nothing; the internal environment is everything."

Healing is accomplished not by attacking the secondary cause, but by eliminating the primary cause of disease. In other words, healing requires cleansing the body's internal cellular environment and restoring its health.

> ॐ
>
> Illness is the expression of an effort by the body to purify and preserve itself. It is not a task aimed at destroying health.

REMEDIES AND THERAPIES

Helping the Body to Heal Itself

If all the health problems occurring in specific regions of the body (local disorders) are a result of the defective state of the body's biological terrain, and if the ability of germs to launch a successful attack is also dependent on those weaknesses, then it is simply good sense for the therapist to focus first and foremost on this internal cellular environment. The unity of disease concept has its correspondence in therapeutic uniqueness: the correction of the biological terrain through purifying it and amending its deficiencies.

The first objective, therefore, is to free the body of toxins and waste. To achieve this goal, it is necessary to completely clear all the body's exits, or organs of filtering and elimination: liver, intestines, kidneys, skin, and respiratory tract. These organs are always working at a slower pace in sick individuals. The wastes that accumulate there, which the organs are unable to expel from the body, are then forced deep into the tissues. The various drainage methods, intended to stimulate the excretory organs, will first seek to rid these organs of their wastes, which then allows them to gradually flush out the rest of the wastes stored in the body.

A person needs to have personally experienced or witnessed a drainage cure to truly appreciate just how much

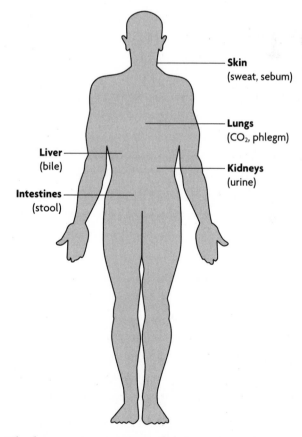

The five excretory organs and their waste products

waste and poison can insidiously collect within the body. Individuals suffering from lethargic intestinal transit are always quite astounded at the quantity of matter that their intestines expel, even after several days of fasting from food, while taking in only water. The strong and nauseating odor of the perspiration of seriously ill individuals is also a well-known phenomenon. By the same token, the deeper color and concentration of urine during a detoxification crisis is always cause for surprise to the novice, as are the many other forms that waste assumes when it is expelled through the skin (pimples, infections, oozing). Despite the often unpleasant nature of these eliminations, they should not be viewed as either discouraging or frightening; it is far preferable to have these wastes outside the body, rather than inside.

Naturopathy calls upon a variety of cleansing methods to stimulate the elimination of toxins. Invariably the techniques are chosen for the particular patient. Depending on the case, the therapist will choose a therapy from medicinal plants, sweat-inducing procedures, enemas, poultices, reflexology, and so forth.

In conjunction with the clearing of the body's avenues of elimination, it is also essential to encourage the emergence of toxins that are embedded in the body. Over time, concentrated wastes not only permeate the bodily fluids, but also become buried in the cellular tissue. These wastes are, of course, much more difficult to eliminate, because they first need to be dislodged before they can be ejected from the depths of the tissues and carried to the excretory organs by bodily fluids. The techniques used for this purpose either encourage a significant increase in the flow of cellular fluids, accelerate circulation, or break down wastes embedded in the tissues into smaller particles that are easier for the body to transport and eliminate. These techniques include fasts, mono diets (limited to a single food), balneotherapy, lymphatic drainage, specific physical exercises, and so forth.

By stimulating the intestines with laxative (elimination-inducing) plants or enemas, encouraging the elimination of urine with diuretic plants, encouraging expectoration with essential oils, and perspiration with hydrotherapy or balneotherapy, the naturopath is doing nothing other than imitating the healing procedures implemented by the body itself. The vital force triggers abundant elimination of waste through the digestive tract (diarrhea, vomiting), kidneys (thick, acidic urine), respiratory tract (mucus), and skin (sweat) to purify the body and restore it to good health. In mimicking this process, natural medicine respects the great truth proclaimed by Hippocrates: "Medicine is the art of imitating the healing procedures of nature."

The second objective of naturopathy is to correct the biological terrain by supplying what it needs to recover its equilibrium, and satisfying its deficiencies. If deficiencies in essential amino acids, minerals, vitamins, and trace elements have a dramatic effect on bodily function, it is simply because our bodies are unable to manufacture them and must get them from the outside.

A body that is given substances it was previously deprived of for a significant length of time will feel reborn and, amazingly, recover all its strength. All the physical and mental functions that had been dulled or lethargic will resume activity, all work left in suspended animation will be put back in motion, and the body will revive. The biological terrain will then be purified much more quickly, and the immune forces will recover their normal strength.

One can satisfy body deficiencies by regular consumption of foods containing the missing substances, or with the help of restoratives like bee or flower pollen, royal jelly, brewer's yeast, sprouts, seaweed, or certain shellfish. The abundance and concentration of vitamins, essential amino acids, trace elements, and minerals in these food supplements support the body's natural vital forces and fill its deficiencies more rapidly.*

~:~

In allopathic medicine the diagnosis of the patient is considered to be the most important point to be resolved, because medical prescriptions will be determined by clues that indicate a specific disease. These clues are revealed by examination of the patient. This kind of therapy looks like a kind of equation: this disease = this medication. Until there is a diagnosis, treatment cannot begin. The patient is therefore placed under observation, which in reality means that the biological terrain will be left to continue to deteriorate until a diagnosable local disorder appears.

It is only then that a course of treatment can be initiated and the correct therapeutic agent chosen to combat the illness.

There is another major inconvenience with this concept of medicine. When a new and unknown disease appears, such as AIDS, the patient is forced to invest all his hope in the day when the disease will be fully identified and a cure manufactured.

Naturopathy does not allow itself to be halted by a "new" and "unknown" disease. All that is new about any illness is the way it manifests a disorder buried in a constricted biological terrain. Even in the absence of a diagnosis in the standard allopathic sense, treatment can begin.

---

*See also the glossary entry for Naturopathy for an outline of techniques used by naturopaths to restore and maintain health.

There is no need for the patient to be placed under observation, to wait while his problems grow worse and hope for the discovery of a cure. The correction (draining wastes and filling deficiencies) can be started at once.

In allopathic medicine the diagnosis is based on the illness; in naturopathy it is based on the patient. It is not so much a diagnosis as it is a health assessment indicating what imbalances need correction. The therapist takes an interest in the patient's lifestyle, organ strength, immune system, deficiencies, and the nature and causes of body fluid congestion.

The therapist is concerned with the total human being—physical, mental, and spiritual—rather than isolated fragments of his or her total being, because the corollary to a fragmentary diagnosis is a fragmentary treatment. Naturopathy strives to realize an in-depth treatment that addresses the profound nature of the illness rather than its superficial manifestations.

⁓

It is worth taking a moment here to ask ourselves what makes a remedy effective. How does it work? Customarily, one has the impression that the remedy encompasses all the healing powers necessary to effect a cure, and that it is the unique active agent. If we define the effectiveness of a remedy by its ability to cause the symptoms of a disease to vanish, this is the way it can seem. But if we consider disease to be a defective state of the body's internal cellular environment, we need to question how a remedy, versatile as it may be, can stimulate the excretory organs, purify the tissues, strengthen the immune system, fill the body's deficiencies, and dissipate local symptoms all by itself.

The remedy does not heal the disease; it helps the patient self-heal. The powers of healing reside within the body. They are the body's vital forces, what the ancients called its medicalizing nature, and what moderns call the immune response. Therefore the conversation is about self-healing, not just healing. No remedy is capable of healing the diseases of a dead person. A corpse lacks the vital, organic force that will be able to stimulate, direct, and support it.

However, it is important to note that naturopathy is not opposed to the use of remedies. It makes use of them, but uniquely, as a supplement to its treatment of the body's deep-rooted issues. Rather than pinning all possibility of a cure on a sole specific remedy, as allopathy does, naturopathy acts on the biological terrain that is responsible for the specific local disorder. Furthermore, because the specific remedies it employs for local disorders are physiological and not chemical, they are accepted into the body's metabolic circuitry, and can be easily used and eliminated by the body. When this is not the case, remedies will only increase the degradation of the biological terrain, creating an effect that is more harmful than beneficial.

It is certainly sometimes necessary to use remedies whose "cure is worse than the illness" when their temporary use makes it possible to get through difficult junctures: an explosion of bacterial activity, intense pain, abrupt weakening of an organ, and so forth. But whereas the use of these remedies should be the exception, it has become the rule. This is why we're witnessing an explosion of iatrogenic diseases, illnesses that are caused by the medications themselves. The rationale that the iatrogenic illness is less serious than the initial disease is not a valid argument for the use of these medications. Local symptoms and disorders may appear less grave, but the degradation of the biological terrain is aggravated even further by the medication-induced toxic overload, prefiguring new diseases.

It is always disconcerting for those who prescribe chemical medication, as well as for those who use it, to see the procedures employed in natural medicine. How can herb teas and tinctures compete with products that have an incomparably higher concentration of active ingredients? How can applications of water, diet, or massage claim to bring about healing where the most powerful medications remain impotent? Here we should recall that the value of a remedy does not reside in itself but in its capacities to aid, support, and stimulate the body's own healing powers.

ॐ

The forces of healing are located inside the body.

The value of a remedy does not reside in itself but in its ability to stimulate these vital forces.

FICTITIOUS HEALING VS. TRUE HEALING

Addressing Causes, Not Just Symptoms

Since illness is rooted in the body's internal cellular environment, healing must transpire on this same level of the biological terrain, and not at the level of the local disorder. Health is not the absence of surface symptoms, but corresponds to a particular state of the body's biological terrain in which the composition of the bodily fluids permits and encourages normal cellular activity. True healing is the kind of healing that restores the biological terrain to its optimum state.

The clearing up of local disorders cannot be considered

to be a healing of the illness if the biological terrain upon which these disorders appeared has not also been changed. Of course the cessation of painful or debilitating local disorders can be hailed as a good thing, but this gain will not last for very long if the root of the illness has not been addressed.

Unless there is change in the status of the bodily fluids, we will experience or witness many relapses, often incorrectly identified by standard medicine as new attacks that will then require new treatments to repress the symptoms. This is a real battle against the seven-headed hydra. Hardly has one local disorder been put down than the vital force will trigger another healing crisis at the same excretory location (known as a relapse) or at another location in the body (a transfer of disease, which is simply a redirection of wastes to another excretory organ).

Multiple attempts by the vital force to purify the body can take place simultaneously at several locations. The unknowing and poorly advised patient will then race from one specialist to the next for treatment of the different local disorders, whereas a single treatment—the correction of the biological terrain—would cause all of them to vanish. Let me repeat, the illness is always one and the same, it only manifests differently depending on where in the body it is located.

Superficial healings obtained locally by treatments targeting the symptoms ultimately fail, because toxins remain buried in the depths of the tissues. The body is thus forced to tolerate an increasingly elevated rate of overloads. The patient seems cured, but his or her biological terrain continues to degrade. In reality, the patient is becoming sicker and sicker.

A real healing can be obtained only by restoring the

norms of the biological terrain, which can be achieved only by purifying it completely. These measures addressing the depths of the body will automatically bring about the disappearance of local disorders—and in a definitive manner—if the errors that created the degradation of the biological terrain are not repeated.

The defined and labeled local disease is only the ultimate culmination of a long process of degradation of the body's internal cellular environment that may have stretched over months or even years, so there should be no illusion of a fast and easy cure by a miraculous remedy. A cure can be obtained only through the implementation of a process that is the reverse of the one that caused the degradation of the biological terrain. All toxins that have entered the body must be eliminated, all deficiencies need to be replenished, and all damaged tissue must repair itself.

In all diseases, but especially in serious diseases, one must fortify oneself with patience and look at the long term. There are no possible shortcuts. The disappearance of a local disorder does not mean that the internal cellular environment has been cleansed from top to bottom. To the contrary, the symptoms can disappear fairly quickly, precisely because they are only the terminal culmination of a deep-rooted disorder. They are like the last drop of water that causes the glass to overflow, or the straw that breaks the camel's back. The most important thing to emphasize here is that it would be a mistake to stop treatment at the point when the local disorder disappears.

Halting one's intake of pharmaceutical medicine as soon as the symptoms have vanished fits into the logic of the medical approach that considers these local symptoms to be the integral disease. This way of doing things cannot be transposed into treatment that will correct the body's biological terrain. Naturopathic treatment should be continued for some time after the symptoms disappear.

The treatment of the biological terrain does not, however, offer protection against new assaults by toxins, or deficiencies in other essential substances. Any change in the patient's lifestyle that was adopted to obtain a cure must be maintained afterward, with some adjustments, lest the same causes recur and prompt the symptoms to reappear. This lifestyle change is the price of true and lasting healing.

The disappearance of local disorders cannot be considered a healing of the disease unless the biological terrain hosting the disorder has also been changed.

THE DIFFERENT STAGES OF DISEASE

From "Not Feeling Well" to Serious Illness

The difference between a benign illness and a serious disease is not a difference of type, but of degree. Fundamentally, all diseases possess an identical nature. But in serious illness, the degree of deterioration of the biological terrain and the scope of the damage it causes are much greater than in more common illnesses. The deficiencies are more pronounced, the overloads more abundant, and the disruption of cellular life more significant. The state of decay in the biological terrain is such that the physical and mental functions of the body are not only restricted or perturbed, they have deviated significantly or stopped completely. How is it possible for living matter to reach such a state of chaos?

As we have seen, diseases do not make a sudden

appearance but are the culmination of a long process. Serious diseases such as cancer, AIDS, or multiple sclerosis do not suddenly strike someone enjoying good health. They constitute the terminal manifestation of a state of defective health that may have been building over many years.

The fact that children, as well as adults, may be stricken by serious illness shows how immensely important it is to avoid fictitious healings that create only the appearance of health, and to concentrate our search on cures that guarantee true health. These alone will permit the transmission of strong, healthy cellular terrain to our descendants.

Disease progresses through three different stages before it becomes a serious and degenerative illness.

First Stage

The first stage is the stage of warning signals, when a person who has been enjoying sound health observes the appearance of minor health problems. These warnings that the person is leaving the ideal state of health may be, for example, a loss of enthusiasm and a lack of pep, temporary indisposition, difficulty recovering after exertion, or even pimples or digestive disorders. The skin may lose its sheen and the hair turn dull and lackluster. All of these are signs that the biological terrain is becoming degraded. The rate of overload is still low during this stage, and these kinds of disorders will disappear quickly if the individual considers them as warning bells and takes appropriate action. In other words, she should scrutinize her lifestyle over the days or weeks preceding the appearance of any health problems to identify what has produced these alterations in her biological terrain.

Has she put a strain on her health from overeating,

consuming toxins, overworked nerves, lack of sleep, or being too sedentary? The biological terrain deteriorates every time the lifestyle exceeds the body's working capacity, or every time the body's physical and mental capacities are diminished for one reason or another and can no longer perform the tasks required of them.

If the patient refuses to listen to the warnings being issued by her body and continues living extravagantly without making any course corrections, the biological terrain will continue to deteriorate. The collection of waste and toxins in this internal cellular environment will go on until it reaches the threshold of tolerance, when a vigorous reaction by the body's vital forces will trigger a health-restoring cleansing crisis.

Second Stage

The second stage, that of acute illness, is reached at this point. Any further possibility of tolerating the rising level of toxins has been exceeded, and all of the body's vital forces are mobilized to expel the excess waste from the body. Depending on the location or form taken by these cleansing crises, allopathic medicine might diagnose the flu, measles, bronchitis, and so on, labeling each of these defensive reactions of the body as diseases in their own right.

In general, acute illnesses are violent and spectacular. The fever accompanying them reveals the intense activity the body deploys to renew itself. This activity is extended all over the body, moreover, and calls on the services of all the excretory organs. The flu, for example, is characterized by abundant secretions from the respiratory tract, intestinal upset, profuse sweating, and waste-laden urine. Acute illnesses are of short duration because the intensity of the effort of organic purification is sufficient to restore order rapidly.

Fever: Why We Heat Up

Fever is a reflection of the body's attempt to defend itself from a biological terrain overloaded with toxins. The acceleration of immune defenses, blood circulation, respiration, and cellular exchanges produces heat and thereby increases body temperature. Fever is, therefore, a manifestation of the body defending itself, which is why it is a common symptom of so many different maladies. It is the body's brilliant way of incinerating and eliminating a large amount of toxins in a short space of time.

Unless the patient's temperature climbs so high that it poses its own risks to the body, breaking a fever will only obstruct the body's defense system.

The confusion at this stage is to mistake the effect for the cause. If these defensive reactions are erroneously perceived as the cause of the disease and not as an effect of the deterioration of the body's internal cellular environment, the therapy will not be directed toward helping the body in its efforts to purify itself, but toward repressing unwelcome and troublesome symptoms. The treatment for the symptoms will halt all efforts of the vital force—in other words, the immune system—and push the toxins deep into the depths of the body. The result will be an increase in the level of toxicity and a decrease in the body's defensive capability.

If the patient, content with the disappearance of his symptoms, resumes his earlier lifestyle, the accumulation of waste will resume. Every new palliative treatment under-taken to repress the efforts of body detoxification (symp-toms) will bring about an increase in wastes and reduce the vital force's ability to respond. Subsequently, at the stage of serious illness, it will be a cause for surprise that the immune system is, for all practical purposes, nonexistent. Yet throughout the patient's entire life, every effort has been made to destroy it.

Third Stage

In the third stage, diseases stop being acute and progress to becoming chronic, or recurring. The overload rate is far too high and the vital force too compromised for any one round of physical cleansing to be sufficient, as is the case with an acute illness. We then see cases of bronchi-tis, eczema, or liver trauma repeating every few months or weeks. Detoxification efforts need to be renewed con-stantly, as they never completely succeed in purifying the internal environment. At this stage, the body absolutely requires outside assistance because its own forces are no longer fully capable of dealing with the congestion of the biological terrain. This support can be provided with cleansing cures, combined with filling the body's deficien-cies, as well as the use of specific physiological remedies. In this way, the biological terrain will recover an almost normal composition and health can be reestablished.

~

Alas, far too often the patient continues to believe a rem-edy is required for each illness, and that each more seri-ous illness demands a stronger remedy. She continues to eliminate the effects without ever removing the causes. The resistance of the biological terrain and the vital force pro-gressively deteriorate.

In the first three stages of the illness, the vital force was still strong enough, to a greater or lesser degree, to expel wastes from the body. But once the fourth stage has been reached, the stage of serious and degenerative disease, this possibility is gone. Wastes and toxins no longer can be expelled properly, and the body's attempt to accommodate itself to their massive presence disrupts its proper functioning. It must fight to survive the highly toxic condition of the biological terrain.

These days, more and more people are coming into the world with such compromised immune systems that, in the evolution of their health problems, they do not even go through the first three typical stages of illness. From birth their bodies have been so overloaded with wastes that no cleansing and regenerative crisis can interrupt the continued degradation of their internal cellular environments.

THE STAGES OF DISEASE

First stage	Warning signals
Second stage	Acute disease
Third stage	Chronic disease
Fourth stage	Degenerative disease

Fourth Stage

During the fourth stage of an illness, what's left of the vital force is still trying to save the life of the patient, but any attempted solutions must take place in the restricted framework of the internal environment, making them increasingly difficult to achieve. Where can the vital force direct the new waves of wastes and toxins relentlessly invading the tissues? How can it continue to protect the cells?

The cells, which should be bathed in nourishing and vivifying pure fluids, are suffocating in fluids saturated with wastes and toxic substances. They are forced to live in a kind of poisoned swamp. In addition they are suffering from a shortage of essential nutrients.

Every kind of physical dysfunction is then possible. Cells become progressively less normal and living matter becomes increasingly disorganized, which is revealed by the destruction of certain kinds of tissue or organs (sclerosis—hardening of a body part, irreversible lesions, deformities); aberrational behavior on the part of the cells, which are no longer subject to the intelligent guidance of the body's vital force (cancer); or by the body's inability to defend itself as an organized unit against microbial and viral assaults (AIDS, various immune deficiency disorders).

At this stage there is much less hope than in previous stages for a remedy or other arbitrary form of intervention that will restore order to the physical chaos reigning in the body. The logical solution is to alter the biological terrain as much as possible in the direction of health, and while waiting for this to be accomplished, support the patient with specific remedies.

The difficulty researchers encounter when attempting to perfect effective remedies against fourth stage diseases stems from the fact that diseases of this nature cannot be cured via shortcuts. It is instead imperative to retrace one's steps while there is still time, and make a focused attempt to cease and amend whatever mistakes have been made against the body's internal cellular environment.

That this is the sole sure means of obtaining remission or a true cure has been abundantly proven by all who have taken this course of action.

❦

Illness goes through three different stages before becoming so serious that it is the terminal manifestation of a state of failing health, one that has been defective for many years.

2

The Causes of Illness
and the Reasons
for Health

ॐ

Because the state of our health is dependent on the state
of our biological terrain, anything capable of causing this
internal cellular environment to deteriorate will inevitably
threaten our overall health.

The more crucial and numerous the factors causing
degradation of the biological terrain, the more it deteriorates and the greater risk we run of falling seriously ill. It
is, therefore, in our best interest to understand these causes
so that we can avoid them. We should not expect to find
these causes in exceptional situations (poisoning or acci-
dental intoxication, for example), but in the habits of our
daily lives.

Our biological terrain is composed of what we ingest as
solid, liquid, or gaseous nourishment (the air we breathe),
as well as everything else that enters the body (food additives, medication, tobacco, and so forth). Every influence to
which our body is subjected becomes encapsulated in our
biological terrain. Simple logic, then, invites us to examine
our lifestyles.

The influence of lifestyle on our health does not always appear obvious because the errors that we make do not always affect us in a way clearly related to what we are doing. These bad habits first bring about changes that eventually grow larger in size—a process that can take months or even years—and become visible on the surface in the form of localized disorders.

Let's take a look at how these mistakes and bad habits break down our biological terrain and make us ill.

> ॐ
>
> All the influences to which our bodies are subjected become encapsulated in our biological terrain, hence the importance of examining our lifestyles.

OVEREATING IN GENERAL

In general, the first and foremost ill effect attributed to eating too much is that it leads to obesity. But eating more than is necessary has a number of other negative repercussions.

Organ Exhaustion

Digestion represents a major task performed by the body. It needs to carry out a series of transformations on the foods ingested, so that they can be absorbed and the valuable nutrients they offer can be made usable by the body.

The force expended for digestion increases with the amount of food consumed. Overeating inevitably leads to general body fatigue. The negative effects of overworking first strike the digestive glands, followed by the heart and the circulatory system that has to transport the excess food products, and finally the excretory organs that are responsible for expelling this vast quantity of waste from the body.

Intestinal Fermentation and Putrefaction

The body's digestive capacity is not limitless. When the amount of food eaten is too large, or when too many different kinds of food are eaten at the same time, the different stages of digestion perform poorly. Food that has not been digested sufficiently will ferment and putrefy in the intestines.

Intestinal fermentation and putrefaction produce a plethora of toxic substances: pyruvic acid, scatol, indole, ptomaine, and so forth. If these substances can be speedily flushed out of the organism, they will cause hardly any damage. But because of the fatigue of the digestive and excretory organs, this is exactly what doesn't happen. This is the way the body poisons itself with toxic substances.

Self-poisoning

Depending on the degree of the intestinal breakdown, the speed of the intestinal transit can be slowed so considerably that fecal material remains inside the intestines for days, or even weeks, causing self-poisoning. The intestinal mucous membranes are attacked and irritated by these unexcreted poisons with which they are now in prolonged contact. Eventually they develop lesions and become porous. From this point, instead of allowing only nutritive substances to flow into the bloodstream, the destroyed mesh of their walls also allows the passage of larger toxic molecules.

By creating a situation that leads to lesions in the intestinal mucous membrane, overeating throws open the doors to intestinal poisons and wastes. As long as the liver can manage to neutralize these wastes, they will not cause the body any undue suffering. But once the anti-toxin function of the liver has been exceeded by the mass of wastes it is receiving on a daily basis, the liver can no longer protect the body and little by little will become completely overrun by these toxins. The patient actually poisons himself with his own wastes.

The Accumulation of Overloads

Even if digestion is functioning perfectly well, overeating will still cause the biological terrain to break down. Indeed, when overeating takes place, the body is receiving more food than it needs. What should it do with the excess nutritive substances?

It can place part of them in reserve, storing them in anticipation of future needs, as it does with fat or glucose. But the body's storage capacities are not unlimited either. When there is an overabundance of any stored substance in the body, even a useful one will become harmful. Just think, for example, of diabetics who suffer from a variety of ailments, all of which can be traced to the poisoning of their body by sugar. Likewise, the excessive fat collected in the tissues of obese individuals will eventually cause them major problems such as slowed circulation and cellular exchange, useless fatigue of the heart and organs, and clogging of the organs.

Instead of storing excess substances, the body also can try to eliminate them. It first needs to break them down into a form the excretory organs will find easy to expel. However, the breaking down of these substances, which would free the body from undesirable overloads, does not take place properly because of the overall slowed pace of bodily functions. Breaking down glucose, for example, does not end with the normal production of easily eliminated water and carbon dioxide, but comes to a halt at an intermediary stage that produces numerous toxic acids (pyruvic acid, succinic acid, fumaric acid, and so on).

Even if the breakdown of excess substances takes place normally, it is still producing toxins. For example, the degradation of proteins inevitably leads to the production of urea and uric acid.

Overeating does not necessarily lead to gaining weight. It can also, without any increase in pounds, congest the body enough to cause significant changes in the composition of bodily fluids.

Excretory Insufficiency

The body's use of food substances always produces waste and toxins. This involves a normal and entirely anticipated process, since the role of the excretory organs (liver, intestines, kidneys, skin, and lungs) is specifically to eliminate these wastes. Of course, the greater the quantity of food consumed, the greater the quantity of wastes that will be produced.

When they exceed the eliminatory capacity of the excretory organs, toxins clog the "filters" and cause congestion in the organs. As elimination becomes unable to take place properly, waste starts collecting in the tissues.

How Does One Overeat?

Practically speaking, there are two different ways in which it is possible to overeat, although they can be combined: eating too often or eating too much at one time.

In addition to their three regular meals, many people take breaks around 10:00 a.m. and 4:00 p.m. to eat snacks. These foods are intended to "just tide me over," but teatime and coffee break snacks are often just as rich as the three main meals of the day. These people are actually eating not just three meals a day but rather five or more! The cakes, cookies, chips, sandwiches, coffee drinks, and candies that are the usual "snack" culprits represent a substantial portion of the daily dietary intake.

In the second kind of overeating it is not necessarily the amount of food that is most important, but its questionable nutritional value. These foods are too rich, with too many calories and too few nutrients.

At mealtime, instead of consuming the recommended 70 percent "light" foods (salads, raw and cooked vegetables, fruits) and 30 percent concentrated foods (meat, cheese, eggs, grains, fatty foods), the proportions are reversed. The core of the meal is formed by meat, often served with fattening, flour-thickened sauces, whereas the portions of fruit and vegetables are extremely limited. Sometimes it seems as if these latter foods are only for decoration.

Overeating is rampant in every strata of the population. Although the real needs of an adult are placed around 2400 calories a day, actual intakes are much higher. The average daily caloric intake in Switzerland is around 3,380 calories, 3,633 calories in France, 3,651 in Belgium, and 3,654 in the United States.

> ৵৽
>
> Overeating wears out the body and overloads it with waste.

OVEREATING SPECIFIC SUBSTANCES

In overeating in general, the subject eats everything in too large a quantity. When there is overconsumption of specific foods, these are cases in which a single kind of food is consumed in quantities higher than the body can properly digest and utilize.

All the problems encountered with general overeating are also problematic in specific foods, but with the addition of the distinct problems specific to the foods being consumed in excess. There are primarily four foods incriminated in this group: sugar, meat, fat, and salt.

Diets Too Heavy in Sugar

The digestion of foods rich in carbohydrates—fruit, grains, bread, potatoes, refined sugar products—provides glucose for fuel, which the body requires in order to function.

In order to be transformed into energy, glucose goes through two metabolic phases: an anaerobic phase (in the absence of oxygen), and an aerobic phase (in the presence of oxygen). During the anaerobic phase, through the action of different enzymes, glucose is transformed successively into citric acid, alpha-ketoglutaric acid, pyruvic acid, succinic acid, fumaric acid, malic acid, oxaloacetic acid, and finally lactic acid. These different acids are called the toxic intermediate metabolites (TIM).

In the subsequent aerobic phase, the TIM are oxidized, thereby releasing the energy the body needs. The residue left by this last transformation is composed of water and carbon dioxide, both of which are eliminated easily by the body.

But when there is excess consumption of carbohydrates, the body receives more glucose than it can possibly transform. Instead of culminating with the production of energy, the breakdown of the glucose is interrupted during one of the stages of the anaerobic phase. Whether it is at the pyruvic acid stage or malic acid stage, the intermediary metabolites are toxic residue that will poison the body.

The presence of TIM deteriorates the biological terrain in numerous ways. Blood and lymph have less liquidity, thereby slowing the rate of circulation and exchange and causing congestion in the organs. The mucous membranes of the organs and the walls of the cells are attacked and injured, which increases their vulnerability. A certain number of biochemical reactions no longer can occur because of the change in the pH, or acid-alkaline balance, of the internal environment. The biological terrain becomes increasingly acidic and the body depletes itself by surrendering its alkaline substances to neutralize the excess acidity.* The more carbohydrates consumed, the greater the deficiency in the vitamins and trace elements required to activate the enzymes involved in the breaking down of glucose, and the more the conversion of glucose runs the risk of being halted during its anaerobic phase, which produces TIM.

Consequently, the glucose from foods that are rich in vitamins and trace elements, such as fruit and whole grains, is metabolized much more effectively than the glucose from foods that have scant amounts of these substances, refined foods for instance. Refined sugars (both white and brown) and grains (white rice, white flour, pasta made from refined flour) are large producers of TIM. And yet, the consumption of foods made from white flour and refined sugar is increasing at an alarming rate. The use of white bread is widespread, and the annual consumption of sugar per capita in the United States has gone from 64 pounds in 1900 to more than 139 pounds. The latter figure includes both refined

---

*For more on this, see the section at the end of the chapter, "The Rupture of the Acid-Alkaline Balance," and my book *The Acid–Alkaline Diet for Optimum Health,* Rochester, Vt.: Healing Arts Press, 2003, Revised second edition 2006.

white sugar (62 pounds) and the high fructose corn syrup (77 pounds) found in almost all processed foods. Sugar consumption in the United States is double the European average.

A heavy carbohydrate diet is especially harmful when it includes too many foods containing refined sugar: candy, chocolate, baked items, preserves, commercial soft drinks (averaging 100 grams, or nearly half a cup, of sugar per liter), and sweetened yogurt (16 grams, or more than 3 teaspoons, of sugar per 100 grams) . . . and let's not forget the sugar we add to coffee and tea.

Diets Too Heavy in Protein

Foods rich in protein, such as meat, fish, cheese, eggs, grains, and beans provide the body with the essential amino acids it needs to grow new replacement cells for those that are worn out. The minimum daily protein requirement for the average individual has been strictly established, and it is not large. For healthy adults it is 0.8 gram per kilogram of body weight, which converts to only about 36 grams of protein for every 100 pounds of body weight. All the excess protein that is ingested still needs to be broken down and eliminated, because the body's capacity for storing amino acids in reserve is practically nil. The breaking down of proteins engenders three kinds of extremely toxic waste: uric acid, ammoniac acid, and ketonic acid. While the body is capable of breaking down ammoniac and ketonic acids into less toxic substances such as urea, which is eliminated through the kidneys and the sweat glands, it has no such ability to neutralize uric acid.

When high protein foods are eaten in too high quantities, the body's capacity to neutralize and eliminate the wastes generated by metabolizing them is quickly exceeded.

The result is ammoniac poisoning and accumulation of uric acid in the tissues.

The overeating of high protein foods is the most serious kind of food overconsumption, because the waste created in metabolizing them is the most toxic type of waste that can be created by food in the body.

Additionally, when these proteins are ingested in the form of animal products, the waste does not come merely from the metabolizing of these proteins. Animal tissue also contains all the metabolic waste generated by an animal when it was still alive; in other words, the animal's uric and ammoniac acids, and so on.

At the beginning of the twentieth century in what is commonly known as the developed world (primarily Western Europe and the United States), the annual consumption of meat per capita was around 90 pounds. A century later this figure has more than doubled to 201 pounds, which is a daily meat consumption of more than half a pound. This figure does not include all the protein consumed in foods such as dairy products, eggs, beans, and grains.

These days, a meal without meat is not considered to be a real meal. Furthermore, many people do not take into account that the meat products eaten as a snack, like salami or hot dogs or beef jerky, also represent an intake of meat. Excessive consumption of protein also can come from overeating cheese, eggs, or beans.

Diets Too Heavy in Fats
Fat plays both a building role and an energetic role in our bodies. Fats can be found in oleaginous foods like nuts and seeds (fat content 35–60%), eggs (11.5%), meat (up to 30% fat), sausages (up to 50%), cream (30%), and butter (81%).

Modern studies have proven the existence of two kinds of fat: saturated and unsaturated fatty acids. Unsaturated fatty acids are of vital importance to the body, and are easily metabolized. Saturated fatty acids are another story, however, as the body finds them difficult to use.

It is the latter that are the first to collect in the body's fat reserves (cellulite, obesity) and which adhere to the walls of the blood vessels (cardiovascular disease). Once established in the tissues, they are extremely difficult to dislodge, break down, and eliminate. It should also be noted that excess carbohydrates are stored in the body in the form of saturated fatty acids.

All foods containing fatty substances are composed of both saturated and unsaturated fatty acids, but their proportion varies from one food to the next. The foods that hold the highest concentrations of saturated fatty acids are of animal origin, but this list also includes palm and coconut oils, which are used to make margarine. However, these kinds of margarine are distinctly different from vegetable margarines that are rich in non-hydrogenated and unsaturated fatty acids and are manufactured from cold-pressed virgin oils.

In their natural form, unsaturated fatty acids, generally of plant origin, produce a beneficial effect on the human body by providing it with vitamin F, also known as the Omega 3 and 6 fatty acids. When they are subjected to overly high temperatures, they are adulterated. For this reason, when cooking, it is better to use a good-quality refined oil (sparingly) than the virgin cold-pressed oils.

Excess consumption of fats often goes hand-in-hand with the overeating of meat. This is not only because meats themselves are rich in fats (beef 20%, veal 11%, ham 30%, salami 35 to 49.5%), but also because they are often cooked in grease and fat, and served with equally fat-laden sauces.

Excess ingestion of fatty substances can also be the result of the excess consumption of dairy products, especially butter, whether on bread or vegetables, in sauces and dips, or used in cooking.

The harmful effects of fats are increased even further when they are overheated. In fact, the carbonization of oils or grease during cooking—primarily in frying, deep-frying, and barbecuing—gives birth to substances that are especially toxic and carcinogenic.

Diets Too Heavy in Salt

The foods we are offered by nature contain very little salt. Plant-based foods contain less than 100 milligrams of salt per 100 grams and animal products contain less than 250 milligrams per 100 grams. The salt that we consume is primarily added to foods as part of their preparation (in bread and cheese, for example), as they are cooked, or when they are eaten at the table.

Salt helps maintain the proper rate of water in the body, which means it contributes to ensuring that there is enough fluid within the cells, blood, lymph, and so forth in order for the body to function properly. One of the properties of salt, in fact, is its ability to retain large amounts of liquid (11 grams of water per 1 gram of salt). Salt also helps maintain good muscle tone and blood pressure.

Too much salt in the tissue leads to retention of more fluid than the body needs. This accumulation of water causes weight gain (in the form of water), creates edemas, and tires the heart because it is forced to circulate a fluid mass much larger than what is necessary. Blood pressure will also increase and continue to increase in proportion to the amount of excess salt in the body. This can bring about a variety of health problems associated with high blood pressure as well as cerebral congestion and heart fatigue. Furthermore, the kidneys, responsible for the elimination of salt, will either be assaulted (resulting in inflammation) or clogged (causing kidney stones) by the amount of salt they need to expel. Also, as salt retains water in the tissues it also retains the toxins being held that may otherwise have been eliminated.

Overconsumption of salt is extremely common today. This can be attributed both to a tendency to add much too much salt to our foods before we eat them and to the overconsumption of highly salted foods such as cheese, cold cuts, chips, salted nuts, canned soups, and ketchup. Salt can even be found in sweet foods such as cakes and cookies.

> ❧
>
> The body cannot digest and properly use excess substances.

STIMULANTS

In addition to the actual food we eat, we regularly consume products we mistakenly consider to be food. These are stimulants like coffee, tea, cocoa, soft drinks, and alcohol. Tobacco is another commonly used stimulant, but no one considers it to be a food.

Stimulants contribute practically no nutritive substances to the body. However, one reason they are so widely consumed is that they give the impression of providing energy.

Because of our unnatural—even anti-natural—habits of life (stress, lack of sleep, and so on), we are always tired and consequently we perpetually attempt to energize ourselves with the aid of stimulants. In reality, the energy that is felt on taking a stimulant is not provided by the stimulant itself but is extracted *from our body's reserves.* The truth is that all stimulants contain numerous toxic substances. In order to protect the organism, the vital force triggers a defensive reaction by accelerating the body's metabolism to neutralize, break down, and eliminate these poisons.

This acceleration of the metabolism is experienced as a jolt of energy from outside, whereas in reality the body is only wearing itself out by being forced to react against repeated poisoning. A truly vicious cycle is established: the more the body is revived by stimulants, the more it exhausts itself; the more exhausted it is, the greater its need for stimulation.

During any exertion, there is wear and tear on the tissues and waste production from the breaking down of fuel used by the cells. When it collects in the tissues, the toxins of fatigue can dangerously overload the body's internal cellular environment, especially if the effort is sustained for a prolonged stretch of time. Fatigue is the signal we are given to interrupt our efforts so as to allow the elimination of wastes these efforts have already generated.

If this purification period represented by rest is not respected, and if, by virtue of stimulants, new forces are extracted from the body's reserves to make the continuation of the effort possible, then new toxins are produced. These will combine with those that have already accumulated, and which were the reason for taking the stimulant. When the body is not granted the rest it needs, it becomes more and more poisoned by its own waste.

This endogenous intoxication within the deep tissue is produced by the toxins of fatigue, and only exacerbated by the intoxication resulting from toxins in the stimulants.

Coffee, Tea, Cocoa, Cola

Beverages made from coffee, tea, cocoa, or cola contain varying proportions of one or more of the three following alkaloids: caffeine, theosphylline, and theobromine. These three elements are soluble in both water and in oil. Consequently, they are able to penetrate any kind of tissue; the protective membrane of the cell, which is fatty, cannot function as a filter against them. The toxic state caused by these alkaloids is, therefore, capable of afflicting even the best-protected tissues, such as those of the nerves and the brain.

The ravages caused by these beverages do not stop there. They also make a significant contribution of tars and oxalic acid. Furthermore, the amount of purine—a substance that gets broken down by the metabolism to become uric acid—contained in these beverages is quite high. Approximately 1 to 2 teaspoons of dried tea (the recommended quantity for one cup) provides as much uric acid to the body as one would get from drinking more than six quarts of milk (approximately 24 glasses).

Alcoholic Beverages

Everyone is familiar with the ravages caused by alcohol, but because we are so used to hearing about them we no longer pay enough attention. People have a tendency to say, "A little alcohol cannot do a body harm," which is essentially true. However the daily consumption of 10 ounces (3 deciliters) a day of wine with 12 percent alcohol by volume will add up to an intake of 4 gallons (15 liters) of pure alcohol in a year's time. The consumption of a liter (most wine bottles are 0.75 liter) of wine with 10 percent alcohol content corresponds to the ingestion of one hundred grams of pure alcohol (nearly one-half cup). Alcohol is not a food but a poison that wears out the liver and irritates and ossifies the tissues.

Tobacco

Although it is constantly repeated that the nicotine, carbon monoxide, cadmium, arsenic, ammonia, and up to 599 legal additives inhaled with every cigarette by smokers—and those around them—are violent toxins, the warnings concerning tobacco poisoning are not taken seriously enough. In fact, there seem to be a large number of people surviving this poisoning, despite daily doses of tobacco higher than what is otherwise believed to be fatal.

It is therefore necessary to specify that the doses commonly cited as fatal are the levels that would be deadly if found *in the blood*. But thanks to the ceaseless efforts of the vital force, the poisons contained in tobacco—just like those of all toxic products of any kind—are rapidly removed from the bloodstream to be eliminated by the excretory organs, if these organs are functioning properly, or buried in the depths of the tissues if they are not. Confronted by such poisoning on a daily basis, the excretory organs are quickly overwhelmed, of course, and the poisons are then deposited out of the bloodstream in the tissues, thereby saving the smoker from poisoning by keeping the blood within norms compatible with life.

But while a quick death is averted, the smoker is still subjected to a slow, widespread poisoning. Throughout the rest of his or her life, the smoker will be beset by numerous disorders that will eventually lead to a slow death through profound degradation of the biological terrain.

> ॐ
>
> When a stimulant is taken, what is felt as a rush of new energy imported from the outside is actually a defense mechanism of the body.

CHEMICAL POISONS

For what is now decades, human beings have been consuming and being poisoned by enormous quantities of chemical ingredients added to their food. This is a critical cause of body fluid congestion.

The different sources of these chemical substances are the following:

Products Used in Farming

Plant fertilizers, as well as the products used to protect crops (insecticides, fungicides, pesticides, herbicides—often twenty to thirty treatments between planting and harvest) partially permeate the tissues of vegetables, fruits, and grains and enter our bodies when we eat the treated foods.

Products Used in Raising Animals

All the medications (antibiotics, vaccines, and so on) and fattening agents (hormones, special diets) given to animals permeate their flesh or their by-products (eggs, milk, dairy products) and ultimately are swallowed by consumers and embedded in their tissues. Only recently, a new threat has emerged—the danger from GMOs, or genetically modified organisms, contained in livestock feed.

Food Additives

These substances are manufactured for the purpose of preserving food products, as well as for making them appear attractive to consumers. They include preservatives, stabilizers, food coloring, flavor enhancers, and so forth. Some of them are perfectly harmless, such as the beet juice that adds red color to fruit yogurt, but others are now recognized as violent poisons. There are several thousand substances used as additives. Although there are only minuscule amounts of each in different foods, there is an estimated annual consumption of several pounds of additives per person each year!

Medications

The majority of medications produced by the pharmaceutical industry are either synthetic products or dangerous chemical substances. Convincing arguments for this are provided on the medications themselves. Simply read the warning labels for the many contraindications and possible side effects. Their risk becomes only more apparent when we see them abruptly pulled from the market for unexpected, disastrous side effects. We also should keep in mind the many iatrogenic diseases discussed earlier.

Household Products

Some of the ingredients in cleaning and beauty products commonly found around the home—detergents, cleansers, shampoos, hair dyes, and so forth—are toxic. Although their toxicity is not extremely high, their regular use is dangerous.

The Products of Pollution

Pollutants contaminate the air, water, and soil. They come from factory smokestacks, automobile exhaust, emissions generated by heating and cooling, and the wastewater created by both homes and industries.

The levels of all of these chemical substances are overseen by official agencies that determine the admissible amount of toxic content in various products and in our environment. Against all normal expectations, toxic or carcinogenic products are not banned outright, but quantities of substances known to be dangerous are regulated so that only very small doses of each can be used. These doses are far below what are deemed to be fatal amounts, and even if they accumulate over time, must not exceed the quantities compatible with life.

You might try to reassure yourself that the experts surely know whether or not the body can tolerate these substances and in what amounts. But a plethora of events and experiments show that they do not really know, and that the human body does not handle being poisoned at all well—even when this chemical poisoning has been approved by the appropriate regulating authorities.

The large-scale usage of additives and chemical medications, which has been accelerating only over the last few decades, is still too recent a phenomenon in terms of human history to allow us to truly measure the long-term effects. The repercussions of toxic poisoning are not always visible immediately. Sometimes lung cancer doesn't declare its presence until thirty or forty years after the smoker takes his first puff.

Furthermore, different experiments seem to show that the appearance of cancerous cells is more rapid when there's a larger daily dose of a carcinogen—in keeping with what one might expect—but surprisingly, that the dose necessary to produce a tumor is practically constant. In other words, it doesn't matter whether the incidents of carcinogen ingestion are close together or spaced further apart, because it is not the quantity contained by the body for a given moment that counts; it is total quantity that has traveled through the body. The effects of each ingested dose, therefore, continue to add up, without any subtraction, over an entire lifetime. Whether the critical level is met by small doses over long periods or just one large dose, it is equally disastrous.

There is yet another concern that needs to be addressed here. While we know very little about the effect of each additive when taken individually, we are even more ignorant about what happens when they combine in our tissues to give birth to completely unknown compounds that might be extremely toxic.

The current multiplication of new forms of serious disease is directly connected to this discreet and insidious chemical poisoning of the body, for which man alone is responsible.

ॐ

The repercussions of a poisonous or toxic state are not always immediately visible.

POOR ELIMINATION

Our bodies are endowed with five organs charged with filtering all the metabolic waste and residue out of the bloodstream in order to expel it from the body. These five excretory organs are the liver, kidneys, intestines, skin, and lungs.

When functioning properly, they are capable of eliminating all the waste produced by ordinary daily life. Even when mistakes have been made, the purity of the biological terrain can still be safeguarded for a certain period of time because the vital force of the body will intensify the filtering and eliminatory work performed by the excretory organs. However, this increased work level cannot be sustained indefinitely.

Sooner or later, the excretory organs will become exhausted and their activity will diminish. If the conditions forcing them to work overtime continue, eventually they will suffer injury and become incapable of functioning normally. It is therefore imperative to rapidly correct all the errors that created this unhealthy condition.

Several figures will allow us to realize the speed with which an organism can become saturated with wastes. The kidneys normally eliminate 25 to 30 grams of urea every twenty-four hours. If they eliminate only 20 grams, that represents a retention of urea of 5 grams a day, adding up to 150 grams (more than five ounces) a month! If, instead of eliminating the 15 grams of salt (NaCl) that are typically absorbed from food every twenty-four hours they expel only 12 grams, this adds up to a retention rate of 90 grams (more than three ounces) of salt in one month.

Of course these figures are not an exact depiction of reality, because the waste that one excretory organ is incapable of eliminating can be eliminated by another, provided the latter's capacities have not been exceeded by overwork as well. But these figures can give us a greater understanding of the quantity of waste that can collect and begin to degrade the state of our internal cellular environment if we do not pay attention to elimination.

So what are the criteria for the proper, healthy functioning of our five excretory organs?

The Liver

The liver filters wastes out of the blood and expels them from the body with the bile. It has an excretory function in addition to its digestive role, inasmuch as it permits the emulsification of fats, an important stage in the digestive process.

Bile insufficiency reveals its presence by overall digestive troubles, abdominal pain, nausea, fermentation, bloating, coating on the tongue, bad breath, and headaches after meals. Another common reaction is feelings of disgust at the mere thought of eating fatty foods such as eggs, fried foods, fat-laden sauces and gravies, and rich pastries; individuals will be incapable of consuming these foods.

The consistency and color of the stool can also reveal this insufficiency. In the absence of bile, the individual is generally constipated and has hard, dry stools that resemble goat dung more than human excrement. The brownish-yellow color of stool is due to the presence of bile pigments. The skin and eyes become yellow when bile is not eliminated properly, because the pigments remain stagnant in the region of the liver, from whence they can easily travel into the bloodstream. A few other revealing symptoms include greasy skin, the propensity to have pimples, and the tendency to suffer inflammation in the respiratory tract.

But even if we are not suffering from any of the problems mentioned above, there is still always the possibility that our liver may be in the midst of becoming deficient because the entire anti-natural lifestyle that is prevalent today contributes to this condition (overeating, chemical poisoning, stress, vaccinations, and so on).

The Intestines

When the intestines are functioning properly, they empty themselves once or twice a day (not necessarily at a set time), and the stools are firm, eliminated easily without straining, and do not have a very strong odor. After one has passed a stool, there should be a feeling of having thoroughly emptied oneself.

But how many people produce only one stool every two or three days, if not less frequently, or have stools that are either dry and hard, or completely loose and repulsive? These individuals often have great trouble evacuating and never have the feeling following a bowel movement that they've emptied themselves completely. This impression is quite accurate—matter is continuing to collect in the intestines, distending and deforming them. Moreover, by fermenting and putrefying while still inside their bodies, this non-eliminated fecal matter starts attacking the mucous membranes of the intestines, which become porous as a result. Instead of being evacuated, some of the wastes are reabsorbed by the damaged mucous membranes and spread throughout the body via the bloodstream.

The Kidneys

The kidneys excrete the wastes they filter out of the blood by diluting them with water. The quantity and characteristics of our urine reveal much about the state of the renal excretory organ. Normally an average 1.5 liters (about 6.5 cups) of urine should be eliminated daily, which means around five to six urinations a day. Because it is carrying waste, urine is colored (golden yellow) and has a distinctive odor.

An individual is suffering from renal insufficiency when the quantity of urine falls below the norm, if she urinates only two to three times a day, or if the urine is too clear and resembles water. In this case the kidneys are certainly eliminating fluid from the body, but not enough waste to give the urine its characteristic yellow color. This observation about color is obviously not valid for people who drink a lot of water—three liters (more than three quarts) a day, for example, as this dilutes the urine and causes it to lose its color.

The Skin

With its sebaceous glands that secrete sebum and its sudoriferous (sweat) glands that secrete perspiration, the skin has a dual elimination system at its disposal. These various glands are quite tiny but numerous. Consequently, they are able to eliminate substantial quantities of waste. During a fever, for example, the skin can perspire quarts of sweat loaded with urea, uric acid, and salt.

Skin that is functioning properly will perspire during times of exertion and when temperatures are high. A person who never perspires or who perspires only from specific locales of the body has an excretory organ that has been practically sealed shut. Because it is incapable of performing the eliminatory duties expected of it, the other excretory organs are forced to work harder. Another sign of poor function is overly dry skin, or, conversely, skin that is too oily or has acne.

The appearance of a pimple or a case of eczema is certainly a defensive reaction of the excretory system, but it is also a sign that eliminations must not be functioning well, because wastes are stagnating in the region of this excretory organ.

The Lungs

Wastes that are eliminated by way of the respiratory tract should first and foremost be of a gaseous nature—carbon dioxide and water vapor. Solid wastes should be extremely rare and primarily consist of dust that has been inhaled and trapped in the filters of the upper respiratory tract. It is not normal to have a constantly runny nose or to be coughing and expectorating. People prone to inflammation in the mucous membranes of the respiratory tract (colds, sinusitis, bronchitis) are showing evidence of congestion of

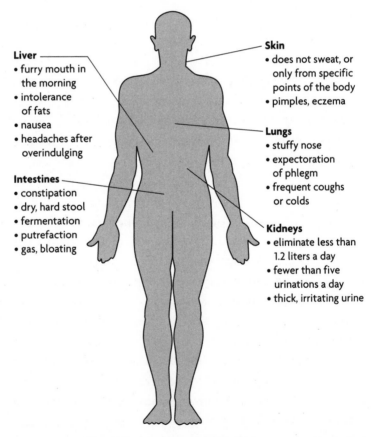

Liver
• furry mouth in the morning
• intolerance of fats
• nausea
• headaches after overindulging

Intestines
• constipation
• dry, hard stool
• fermentation
• putrefaction
• gas, bloating

Skin
• does not sweat, or only from specific points of the body
• pimples, eczema

Lungs
• stuffy nose
• expectoration of phlegm
• frequent coughs or colds

Kidneys
• eliminate less than 1.2 liters a day
• fewer than five urinations a day
• thick, irritating urine

Signs of excretory organ weakness

the biological terrain and overworked excretory organs.

The inhalation and exhalation of air should be regular, deep, and easily adapted to a change in rhythm during intense periods of exertion. Someone who runs out of breath too easily, even during slight exertion, or who is often gasping for air or frequently needs to spit out colloidal waste, has an overloaded pulmonary excretory organ wherein gaseous exchanges are not taking place properly.

〜

Expulsion of waste from the body is not the sole task performed by the excretory organs. They must first filter and extract these wastes from the bloodstream, then prepare them in a way that allows them to leave the body without injuring the tissues.

Each excretory organ filters and eliminates specific wastes. When one of these organs can no longer manage to eliminate all the wastes presented by the body, another excretory organ steps in and eases its workload. For example, colloidal wastes that the liver is incapable of filtering can be expelled through the sebaceous glands or respiratory tract.

A system of mutual aid, therefore, exists between the excretory organs and allows them to protect the purity of the biological terrain by ensuring that the essential task of eliminating waste continues to take place. Of course this system can only function as long as the assisting excretory organs are not themselves overworked. If this is the case, deep and rapid congestion of the body will occur.

It is easy to see that the deficiency of one excretory organ does not lead directly to serious illness. But the chronic insufficiency of one or several of these organs will certainly lead to a state of poor health eventually, because of the progressive saturation of the biological terrain with wastes. Those suffering from serious, or big illnesses are all "small eliminators."

> ❧
> Big illness patients are all "small eliminators."

A SEDENTARY LIFESTYLE

In addition to weakened muscles and organs, a sedentary lifestyle causes decreased oxygenation, slowed metabolism of food intake, and poor elimination of toxins.

Our ancestors were much more physically active than we are today, simply out of necessity. Elevators, automobiles, supermarkets and the like have created an "easy life" that's not so easy on our bodies. Our motor capacities are underutilized, either because of jobs that require us to remain seated, our use of motor vehicles to travel rather than walk even short distances, the absence of physical activity during leisure time, or all of the above.

The lack of time that often serves as a pretext for not walking, taking the stairs, or preparing foods manually is just that—a pretext because time that is saved in this way is used by most people in sedentary pursuits, like sitting for hours in front of the television or computer, or traveling long distances to get to . . . the gym.

DEFICIENCIES

The body does not hold within its tissues all the nutritive substances it will need over the course of a lifetime. It is, therefore, necessarily dependent on what is provided by sources outside the body. Our food should regularly bring us sufficient quantities of all the nutrients (amino acids, carbohydrates, fats, minerals, vitamins, and so forth) that are essential for the formation and maintenance of our organs as well as their functioning.

Once the body is deprived of one of these nutrients, its functioning is disrupted; the first sign is the slowing of one or more body functions. Subsequently, if the deficiency lasts too long, certain physical and mental functions can grind to a halt. If it remains uncorrected, death will eventually ensue. For example, depending on what substances the body lacks, tissues will no longer be repaired, the resistance of the mucous membranes diminishes, there is a loss of muscle tone, enzyme activity is reduced, secretions stop, the blood becomes thinner, and white blood cells lose their defensive ability.

In illnesses caused by deficiencies, nothing can halt the evolution of the disorder and the degradation of the biological terrain other than restoring an adequate supply of the missing substance. As long as this substance remains absent, the body will continue to go downhill. Because the body is totally dependent on the missing nutrient, no medicine is capable of taking its place. Just as the solution to this problem is simple—the ingestion of several milligrams of vitamins, for example—a disorder can remain serious so long as the deficiency remains unaddressed.

Even a deficiency of a single nutrient can have catastrophic consequences. In fact, nutrients work interdependently with one another. The absence of just one can, therefore, render the utilization of the others completely ineffective, and like a chain reaction, create a state of multiple deficiencies.

Although we live in an era of abundance, it is much easier to experience deficiencies of this nature than one might think. It might be a deficiency of supply (the foods ingested by the body do not contain all the necessary nutrients), or it could be a deficiency of utilization (the nutrients are supplied to the body but the body is unable to make use of them).

Deficiencies of Supply

In the simplest case, foods containing the missing substance are not being eaten by the individual. In the past, this was a common occurrence for inhabitants of extremely isolated regions that had a limited number of foods at their disposal. Today, deficiencies of supply are more likely to be due to a deliberate—but erroneous—eating choice. Many people, perhaps because they have been misinformed or have not grasped the entire picture, totally banish one food or entire food category from their diets and practice skewed diets that lead directly to the various diseases caused by deficiencies. Some people indiscriminatingly eliminate all fat from their diets after having read somewhere that fats were implicated in cardiovascular disease. Others avoid eating a certain fruit for fear of being poisoned by pesticides, and so on.

Diets that are practiced for philosophical or aesthetic reasons can also create serious deficiencies, if these individuals do not take into consideration the physiological imperatives of the body.

Another very common cause for deficiencies of supply today arises from the fact that our food no longer contains all the nutrients it should. These elements have been removed by various procedures that alter the food's outer appearance or increase its shelf life. Perhaps grains have been refined, a process that makes it possible to obtain extremely white flour, but which deprives the consumer of precious nutrients that are located in the part of the grain that gets discarded in the refining process. Vegetable and plant oils are also subjected to a series of mechanical, caloric, and chemical transformations that cause them to lose their vitamins and trace elements. The same holds true for refined sugar, which, stripped of all living elements, can be preserved almost indefinitely. Additionally, the depletion of soil and inadequate farming or livestock-raising methods is likely to result in a sharp drop in the nutrient content of foods, as is the drying of fruits at high temperatures, eating only cooked foods, and throwing away the cooking water.

A special word needs to be said concerning water. Of all the substances our bodies need, water is a top priority inasmuch as our bodies primarily consist of fluids. Daily intake of sufficient water is, therefore, essential. The reality is that many people are not drinking enough water; their daily consumption is clearly below the 2 liters, or slightly more than half a gallon, that their bodies require every day. This shortage of water creates a state of chronic tissue dehydration that hampers the body's normal functioning.*

Deficiencies of Utilization

This kind of deficiency is caused when the body finds it impossible to utilize some of the nutrients with which it has been provided.

This could be either because the nutrients were destroyed in the intestines before they could be absorbed into the bloodstream by toxic substances resulting from intestinal fermentation and putrefaction, or because the biological terrain is so saturated with wastes that exchanges

---

*For more on this see my book *The Water Prescription,* Rochester, Vt.: Healing Arts Press, 2006.

are occurring poorly. In either case the result is the same: the nutrients don't reach the area of the body where they can be used.

Numerous chemical substances from additives, pollution, and pharmaceutical medication have an inhibiting effect on vitamins and trace elements. When this occurs, they can be described as anti-vitamins, or chelators of trace elements. The nutrients are present in the body but have been rendered inactive, or even destroyed, by chemical pollution. The individual suffering from deficiencies can supply her body with all the proper nutrition it needs, but in vain; the consumption of these inhibitors creates a state of deficiency in the body, in addition to other toxic effects.

The simple consumption of stimulants causes deficiencies because their use demands more nutrients that will allow the body to neutralize the poisons of the stimulants. The consumption of tobacco increases the body's need for vitamin C, alcohol for vitamin B, and so forth. It is important to note that deficiencies in vitamin C reduce the body's capacity to defend itself, and deficiencies in vitamin B disrupt the nervous system and encourage clogging of body fluids because of the poor utilization of food that results.

Another reason why the body finds itself incapable of benefiting from the nutrients it is supplied stems from the fact that they are removed before it can put them to use. In fact, numerous deficient foods, such as refined sugar, white flour, and refined oils, as well as all the food products prepared with them, are known as "vitamin thieves." Because these foods are incomplete they no longer carry the enzymes, vitamins, and catalytic metals required to digest them. In order to make the digestive breakdown of these deficient foods possible, these vital substances will be pilfered from the body. Refined and processed foods, even before they give the body whatever nutritive substances they might still carry, are desecrating what is already there.

When incomplete and deficient foods like these are consumed on a regular basis, the body's reserves end up being pillaged, and serious deficiencies can be established.

> ❧
>
> Once the body has been deprived of any one essential nutrient, its functioning will be disturbed.

THE RUPTURE OF THE ACID-ALKALINE BALANCE

Our bodies function best when the acidic and alkaline substances that enter into the composition of tissues and bodily fluids are present in equal quantities—what we call the acid-alkaline balance.

A Precarious Balance

The body contains both acid and alkaline substances, and the balance between them is critical to our good health. This balance—the degree of acidity or alkalinity in the body—is measured as pH. The normal pH of blood, and of the biological terrain in general, is 7.39. When there is movement away from this ideal pH, frequently caused by our acid-producing diet and lifestyle, the bodily terrain becomes highly susceptible to disease.

Any disruption of this balance will lead to illness. The most common rupture, extremely widespread at present, is the one characterized by a disproportionate amount of acid in the internal cellular environment, or acidosis. The health problems that this can cause are quite varied: chronic fatigue, stress, excessive nervousness, depression, rheumatic disorders, tendinitis, eczema, tooth decay, and so forth.

How are these disorders formed? Acids have virulent properties that irritate the tissues and can go on to cause inflammations, for example of the joints and tendons. In order to defend itself, the body seeks to neutralize the excess acid with the help of its buffer system. To do this, it steals the alkaline minerals found in the blood and tissues. In times of heavy demand or regular withdrawals, the organs and tissues lose their mineral content and become weaker and more fragile (dental cavities, eczema, nervous fragility . . .). Furthermore, an acidic biological terrain is an environment that provides unfavorable working conditions for enzymes, those "little workers" responsible for all the biochemical transformations that take place in the body. Energy production, tissue regeneration, and cellular exchanges all diminish and are replaced by chronic fatigue, depression, reduced defenses, and a marked loss of enthusiasm.

The principle cause for the rupture of the acid-alkaline balance toward acidity is dietary. The proportion of acidifying food (meat, flour, fat, refined sugar) we consume is generally much higher than that of alkaline food (salad greens, raw and cooked vegetables, potatoes, almonds, bananas). Because it is receiving a much greater quantity of acids on a daily basis than it is alkaline substances, it is a big challenge for the body to neutralize the excess acid. It is therefore obliged to pillage its alkaline reserves from the tissues, with all the unhealthy consequences this theft entails. Usually the body is unsuccessful at reestablishing a perfectly normal pH and must live with this excess acid, which creates a chronic state of recurring disease due to acidosis.

The other causes of acidity are the consumption of stimulants, poor elimination of acids by the skin and kidneys, vitamin deficiencies, and lack of oxygenation. In addition, a negative mental attitude (anxiety, aggressiveness, bitterness, and so forth) will disrupt the metabolism and engender more production of acid by the body. Insufficient sleep and overwork will produce acids as well.

Summary: The Causes of Acidification of the Biological Terrain

- Excess of acidifying and acidic foods and beverages
- Insufficient alkalizing foods
- Under-oxygenation
- Vitamin deficiencies
- Poor elimination by skin and kidneys
- Stress
- Negative mental attitude

As we have ascertained, the major causes for degradation of the biological terrain and those for the formation of an acidic biological terrain are the same. There are, however, several different kinds of biological terrain degradation, of which acidification is just one. It is extremely widespread, because many people have trouble from the outset metabolizing acid, and the excessive quantity of acids consumed in the typical diet rapidly exceeds the body's ability to deal with them.

One means of determining if your biological terrain is acidic is to measure your urinary pH with the help of litmus paper. The normal acid content of the urine is the same as that of the entire body, which we have seen is a pH of around 7. When a person's lifestyle and diet is acidifying,

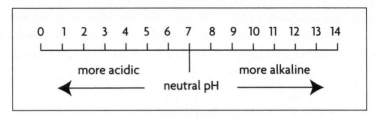

The pH scale

more acids will be eliminated through urination, which will lower its pH to around 6 or 5.

NEGATIVE MENTAL ATTITUDE

Everyone has personally experienced the influence of mental attitude on the body's functioning. The simple nervous anticipation experienced before exams is enough to cause all sorts of disruptions—loss of the desire to eat, sweating, accelerated heartbeat, trembling hands, upset stomach and other intestinal problems, and the persistent desire to urinate. A quarrel that breaks out during the middle of a meal can also be the cause of indigestion. Moreover, grievances can cause loss of appetite, worries can prevent sleep, and so on.

Also, who doesn't know people with liver complaints (hepatics) who experience a liver crisis (nausea, indigestion, vomiting) over the smallest worry and asthmatics who have an attack whenever something upsets them? There are also those who regularly get sick on Monday mornings—both adults in the workforce and schoolchildren—from dread about the week looming ahead.

If the episodes of our mental life, limited in time like the examples just mentioned, can momentarily overwhelm various bodily functions, how much worse are the disorders engendered in someone who agonizes perpetually about everything, dwells on dark thoughts, is easily depressed, fears falling seriously ill, is impatient with those around him, attacks his neighbors, and explodes in rage over the merest trifle?

It would be wrong to think that we are unable to do anything about our individual fortunes and are simply the victims of events. In fact, what is most important is not the situation we are experiencing, but *our attitude* toward it. Some people get irritated at the slightest thing, whereas others are capable of keeping their calm even in the most stressful circumstances.

Two people experiencing the same situation in which both are involved equally—following the death of someone close to both of them, for example—can react in totally different ways. One may be completely stricken by it and fall into a slow decline, whereas the other, although profoundly shaken, will get a grip on his or her feelings and, full of enthusiasm, find new meaning in life.

The power of our attitude and thoughts over events is also revealed by the fact that just to *imagine* an unpleasant situation is enough to cause a change in bodily functioning. The simple mention of forthcoming exams, even weeks in advance, can create anxiety and tie one's stomach into knots. Thoughts of violence and hatred are capable of creating tension even if the person against whom these violent thoughts are directed is absent. Likewise, the joy inspired by an anticipated visit can work positive changes on the overall state of a patient's health.

The influence of thoughts is such that, up to a certain point, even life and death are dependent on them. The will to live of certain seriously ill individuals or accident victims can help them to rise above absolutely desperate situations.

On the other hand, sick or injured people who "give up" or "just let everything drop" sometimes die from disorders that are quite within the scope of therapeutic healing methods.

Because the attitude of the patient has such profound influence on his or her illness, it is clear that the therapist guiding the treatment of these individuals, even when their problems are quite serious, should never diminish the mental aspect of the question as a minor matter while concentrating solely on the material and physical aspects of the patient's case. The psyche exerts its influence on the physical at all times. Just as a negative attitude can increase the serious nature of health problems or hamper their treatment, a positive attitude can lay the groundwork for improvement.

But how, in concrete terms, does a negative attitude cause the state of the biological terrain to deteriorate? Our thoughts and the feelings they engender alter the normal functioning of our organs by means of the sympathetic nervous system and the endocrine glands.

The sympathetic nervous system, which is a part of the autonomic nervous system, regulates unconscious body functions such as salivation, perspiration, air flow to the lungs, and so on. It acts on our body's organs by slowing or accelerating their function, adapting their activity at every moment to the constantly changing needs of daily life. For example, when we need to confront a danger, the digestive functions are inhibited because they are useless as a means of defending ourselves.

Once the danger has passed, the autonomic nervous system slows the circulatory and respiratory functions and stimulates the digestive function so that any interrupted digestion can continue.

But when a person has an erroneous attitude toward life that puts her in a state of constant tension, her digestive functions, to borrow the preceding example, are in a state of chronic indigestion, which is a huge producer of wastes and toxins that contribute to the deterioration of the biological terrain.

Depending on the responses of the sympathetic nervous system to the requests made of it, other changes can occur: elimination will be poor if the excretory organs are permanently inhibited, or there could be a problem with oxidation if it is the respiratory system whose activity is constrained, and so forth.

The endocrine glands, including the thyroid, adrenal glands, and so on, will become disrupted in the same way as the sympathetic nervous system. For example, fear stimulates the release of adrenaline by the adrenal glands, constant irritation and agitation accelerate thyroid function, and so forth. Hormonal secretions also affect the functioning of the organs, and can cause poor digestion or elimination, or a slowing of circulation that will bring about the deterioration of the internal cellular environment.

The influence of mental life over physical health can be subtle, but the fact remains that it is of fundamental importance. More than any other unbalancing factor that asks us to initiate change in our lifestyle, this one demands—if one really wants to be truly cured—profound self-transformation.

❧

The influence of our thoughts is such that, up to a certain point, life and death depend on them.

3

Naturopathy in Practice

---

*Correcting and Balancing
the Internal Cellular
Environment*

ༀ

The first question to leap into the mind of every person in good health who has grasped the importance of the state of the internal cellular environment will be, "What can I do to maintain this state?"

For those suffering from poor health, whose bodies are already overloaded with toxins and deficiencies of essential nutrients, the question obviously will have to be rephrased to, "What can I do to correct my biological terrain?"

In both cases the guiding principles for maintaining or repairing the biological terrain remain identical. The manner of applying them, however, varies enormously from one patient to the next, and from one stage of illness to the next. The advice provided here will necessarily confine itself to introducing and explaining the guiding principles. They can be adopted to great benefit whether someone is sick or enjoying good health. However, they do not suffice in any case for constituting the treatment, properly speaking, of people stricken by serious disease. It is imperative that individuals in this situation seek the help of a qualified medical practitioner. In fact, precisely adjusting the advocated methods to the health needs of every individual, and changing them in accordance with each person's overall state, is an art. Furthermore, the correction of the biological terrain of individuals suffering from serious disease involves a much stricter and more intensive application of the principles presented here.

The guideline for repairing the body's internal cellular environment was given to us by Hippocrates: "Treatment should aim at opposing the cause of the disease and not allowing it to persist." Since illness results from the degradation of the biological terrain by the collection of waste and deficiency of nutrients, the logical treatment would consist of:

- causing those wastes present in the body to be removed,
- preventing new wastes from entering,
- and filling deficiencies.

This approach, like the methods for draining overloads or filling deficiencies, is astonishingly simple. The knee-jerk reaction of the twenty-first-century human being, accustomed to much more sophisticated procedures, will be to doubt the effectiveness of these methods. But they truly are effective because they are based entirely on conformity to natural laws and physiological imperatives. This approach follows the direction of these laws and supports them.

> ॐ
>
> "Treatment should aim at opposing the cause of the disease." —Hippocrates

SHUTTING OFF THE SOURCE OF OVERLOADS

Draining wastes out of the body will not lead to any positive result if, at the same time, other toxins are still being allowed to enter. Over the course of a normal day, new wastes are able to enter our bodies because of our detrimental life habits. If we can correct these bad habits, only one front remains to be conquered. All the body will have to do is eliminate the old, accumulated wastes. It is, therefore, fundamentally important to shut off the perpetual source of new overloads and monitor what we consume.

The regulation of which foods are supplied to the body will of course be more meticulous and precise for someone seriously ill than for someone suffering a minor disorder. When the diet is constantly being adjusted to be in tune with the digestive and excretory capacities of the body, a kind of status quo will be reached. The rate of excess substances does not rise and the organs are never overworked. The strength that is saved in this way is then available for the healing process.

Regulating Quantities

In our era of abundance and chronic overeating, regulating the quantity of food ingested generally means reducing it. But eating less is in no way synonymous with always being hungry and following draconian diets. In accordance with the famous maxim, "You should eat to live, not live to eat," quantitatively regulating your diet merely means that you eat only what your body needs.

If the overeating is due to eating meals that are too big, steps should be taken to make them more modest, either by pure strength of will, preparing smaller quantities, or replacing concentrated foods (meats, fried foods, flour-based foods) with foods of little concentration (vegetables, salads, raw food, fruit).

The overeating we see today is partially due to the poor nutritive quality of our foods. We are instinctively driven to eat more in an attempt to obtain the minerals and vitamins our bodies need but cannot find in the refined foods we offer it. By eating whole foods, and therefore increasing the value of what we ingest, we inevitably will reduce the quantity of food we eat.

Chewing food more thoroughly and for a longer time also helps to reduce the quantity of food ingested. The impression of being full is partially established when the taste buds are saturated with impressions.

Overeating may also be due to an excess amount of snacking between meals. In this case, it's important to be on the lookout primarily for sugar intake. The hunger felt between meals is most often caused by a lack of glucose in the blood. This can be remedied by eating sweet foods (fresh or dried fruit, honey) at the same time as proteins, for example cottage cheese or yogurt. The carbohydrate-protein combination interrupts and stabilizes the use of sugars by the body and makes it possible to maintain normal glycemia, or sugar levels, between meals. Refined sugars in their various forms (chocolates, candies, desserts) are to be avoided at all costs because they encourage the hypoglycemic crises that arouse hunger pangs.

Regulating Quality

Out of ignorance, incomplete information, or thoughtless habit, many people follow irrational and unhealthy diets. Often we consume far too much of one kind of food or totally neglect another. For example, meat is present at every meal but no fruit is eaten at all throughout the day.

The foods eaten excessively in error are primarily meat, refined sugar, fat, and salt:

- With respect to meat, a person will feel much better by consuming this food only once a day, or even better, every two days. If one is sick, it's best to abstain from meat completely for a certain period. Fish is generally less loaded with toxins than meat. It is, therefore, a viable and valuable substitute.

  Total elimination of meat from the diet is only warranted for those suffering from serious disease. Their risk of deficiency is practically nonexistent since meat is extremely low in vitamins and minerals, and the sole valuable nutrient they supply—protein— can be found in many other foods.

- The need for sugar or sweet foods is a legitimate one inasmuch as carbohydrates are an essential fuel supplying energy to the body. But why choose refined sugar, a fuel that makes us sick through demineralization and acidification, when there are others such as fruits and honey that contribute to our good health?

  Individuals suffering from serious diseases should abstain completely from sweets and other food containing refined sugar. This alone will bring about huge health improvements, and would also be beneficial for those with no symptoms.

- Determining the best fats to consume depends on the way they will be prepared and eaten. When cooking, it is best to use a good-quality refined oil (but sparingly!) because they don't adulterate at high temperatures as cold-pressed, virgin oils do. To eat on bread, real butter in small quantities is fine as are vegetable margarines rich in unsaturated fatty acids. For salad dressings, use cold-pressed virgin oils and not refined oils.

- The daily salt requirement is somewhere between 3 and 5 grams. In actual practice, we easily consume much more than that—with some people ingesting as much as 12 to 15 grams a day, three to four times more than the body needs.

  To avoid too much salt in one's diet, first eliminate the "fake" foods that are so high in salt such as chips and salted peanuts. These are not real foods; they are food products that have been manufactured solely to appeal to people's taste buds. Then work toward reducing the salt added during cooking and refrain from adding any extra salt to foods once they reach the dining room table. This will allow for discovery of the true taste of these foods, which is all too often replaced by the taste of salt.

An unbalanced diet can also be caused by the absence of certain foods. Often the deficiency of one food will bring about the excessive consumption of another. The absence of vegetables at a meal will compel the diner to eat more pasta or rice. The food most often absent from the table is fruit, closely followed by vegetables.

For the qualitative regulation of food, we again turn to Hippocrates: "We should reduce what is in excess and add what is lacking."

Eliminating Stimulants

Shutting off the source of overloads also means eliminating all the stimulants in widespread use by people who give little thought to the poisons they contain, and against which the body must fight to render them harmless. In addition, stimulants interfere with the ability to get the hours or quality of sleep required to maintain a healthy body.

When this problem is pointed out to them, consumers of stimulants immediately ask, "Do I really need to do without my morning coffee?" or "Is *one* glass of wine bad for my health?" No, a cup of coffee or a glass of wine is not bad for someone in good health. On the other hand, both are definitively not good for someone who is ill. Furthermore, it is generally not a question of one cup or one glass, but several.

In addition to the well-known ill effects of stimulants like tobacco, alcohol, coffee, and tea, the sleep disruption they can cause is acidifying to the body. Their elimination from the diet will benefit anyone, and is an absolute necessity in cases of serious illness.

However, the weaning period must be handled delicately to prevent any disruption of the already enfeebled bodily functions by abruptly putting the patient in a state of sharp withdrawal. Achieving a dependency-free state should be done as quickly as possible, but gently and gradually so that the body can become accustomed to it without incurring too much disturbance in those functions that have been dependent on habitual stimulation.

Eliminating Chemical Pollution in Food and Medication

Ill individuals are poisoned by waste; their bodies are extremely sensitive to any new form of poisoning, and they will have great difficulty fighting it. Since the body is already working overtime to process accumulated toxins, it is essential to eliminate all possible causes for additional struggle by avoiding any food that contains chemical poison. As much as possible, the ill should eat only food that doesn't contain any dangerous additives: organically grown grains, fruits, and vegetables; and animal products from healthy animals raised in a wholesome environment.

Chemical "medication" is another cause of poison in the body. Sometimes medication is essential, but more often than not it is taken in excess or ill-advisedly. Why not use natural remedies (plants, homeopathic preparations, and so forth) that the body can tolerate easily and which are incontestably effective? All the daily aches, pains, and minor sicknesses can be treated with these remedies. Chemical tranquilizers, pain relievers, and sleep aids often can be replaced by plant-based remedies. More importantly, the practitioner can combine a natural anti-symptom treatment with a treatment targeting the causes of the symptoms.

When food intake has been adjusted to match the body's digestive and excretory capacities, the organs are no longer overworked. The body forces that are preserved in this way are then available for use by the body's healing process.

ELIMINATING TOXINS

When the biological terrain is overloaded with toxins, when the organs are congested and the blood is polluted, when tissues are poisoned and the cells are asphyxiated by wastes, there is only one way to begin to restore the body to health: cleanse it.

An individual truly needs to personally experience a body-cleansing cure to fully appreciate the considerable size that a mass of toxins collecting in one body can assume, and also to appreciate how getting rid of them produces such remarkable health improvement.

The "exit doors" that need to be cleared to allow the toxins to leave are the excretory organs: liver, intestines, kidneys, skin, and lungs. They provide the necessary passageways leading out of the body, and are also responsible for filtering wastes out of the bloodstream.

By stimulating the excretory organs, one is also stimulating the elimination of the wastes that have collected in these organs, thereby encouraging the purification of the blood. But this is not enough to really cleanse the body thoroughly. The great mass of wastes is not found in the bloodstream but has become embedded in the depths of the tissues. These wastes will need to be dislodged from the tissues so that they can make their way into the bloodstream, which in turn will carry them to the excretory organs. To dislodge these toxins permeating the tissues, it is necessary to turn to various methods that differ from those used to stimulate the excretory organs. These methods are used to ensure the removal of the encrusted toxins.

In the application of cleansing cures, these two points have to follow one another in order: The exit doors from the body have to be opened before efforts to dislodge the layers of deeply buried toxins can begin. If one proceeds in the opposite order, or takes both steps simultaneously, the dislodged toxins will arrive in a mass too huge to be processed by the insufficiently opened excretory organs. It is preferable to eliminate all surface toxins before initiating any efforts to excavate toxins buried in the tissues.

Opening the Excretory Organs

There are numerous methods for opening the excretory organs and increasing the elimination rhythm. Those listed here are the most effective and easiest for general application.

The stimulation of the excretory organs can be expedited beautifully by medicinal herbs, if the correct dosage is used. Too weak a dose will not provide sufficient stimulation to the excretory organs, and doses that are too strong will trigger violent reactions that irritate and exhaust these organs. The best way to find the optimal dose without too much difficulty is by starting with weak doses, then gradually increasing the dose every day. One should stop at the dose just below the level that begins to unleash violent reactions.

The several plants or preparations discussed in the following pages, along with instructions for using them, will allow you to put them to work immediately, but this is by no means an exhaustive list. It goes without saying that other plants or preparations can be used with equal success.

When taking drainers—products that encourage the drainage of toxins from the body by stimulating the function of the excretory organs—the patient should be able to objectively observe an increase in elimination of toxins; for example, urine is darker because it is more charged with wastes, and the intestines are emptying properly.

Since the clogging of the body takes place over a span of years, it is important not to nurture false hopes that a draining lasting several days will be enough to unclog and purify the internal cellular environment. Drainage cures, well-adapted to the patient's capacity, should be pursued for several months. When confronted with the length of time these cures require, some patients will worry about becoming dependent on the medicinal herbs they are using, and be hesitant about taking them over a sustained period of time. On the contrary, in their efforts to avoid a potential dependency on these plants, which is an illusory fear, they are only making themselves more dependent on their toxins!

At the start of a cleanse, the various excretory organs will be opened successively to avoid overworking the body. In the next phase they will be stimulated simultaneously, if the patient's health permits. If not, they should be stimulated in alternation, with treatments lasting three to four weeks. Some drainers work on only one excretory organ. For example, hepatics and renal drainers target the liver and kidneys, respectively. When a drainer works on several excretory organs, it is called a depurative.

Drainage of the Liver

If we had to select only one organ to stimulate, it certainly would be the liver. The sound functioning of the entire body is dependent on this organ's healthy functioning. It plays a key role in all vital functions. Not only does it filter and eliminate wastes, but it also neutralizes and destroys poisons and toxins, carcinogenic substances, and germs.

To function properly, the liver requires heat. The liver's optimum working temperature is 102–104°F (39–40°C), thus it operates at a temperature that is higher than that of the rest of the body. Simply sending heat to the liver encourages its proper functioning. One easy solution is to place a hot water bottle on the body near the liver for around ten to thirty minutes, three times a day, generally after a meal. One should not be misled by the simplicity of this procedure. Its amazing effectiveness results from the fact that it works in conjunction with the principles of nature.

There are three plants that stimulate the liver quite well: dandelion, black radish, and rosemary.

- Dandelion (*Taraxum officinalis*) as a mother tincture (maceration of a medicinal herb in ten times its weight in alcohol): 10–50 drops, three times a day with water before meals.
- Black Radish (*Raphanus niger*) in tablets: 1–3 tablets depending on the manufacturer, three times a day with water before meals.
- Rosemary (*Rosmarinus officinalis*): 1 teaspoon of leaves per cup, steeped for 10 minutes, three cups a day before meals.

There are also numerous commercial herb teas indicated as "for the liver and gallbladder," "hepatic depurative herb tea," or some such variation.

Drainage of the Intestines

Together, the small and large intestines form a tube that is approximately 23 feet long and 1 to 3 inches in diameter (7 meters in length, 3–8 centimeters diameter). The intestines can contain an enormous mass of stagnating fecal matter. Draining them means getting rid of this mass that, as a rule, is fermenting and putrefying, thus serving as the starting point for countless infections brought about by the degeneration and mutation of the intestinal flora. This also encourages intestinal disassimilation, the process by which toxins pass through the 1968 square feet or 600 square meters of surface area within the intestinal mucous membranes. The intestines, like all the excretory organs, filter the blood that passes through their tissues to remove the wastes. These wastes are then eliminated with the fecal matter.

A sufficient quantity of roughage (vegetable fiber) is essential for filling the intestine and stimulating its peristalsis. Increased and regular consumption of raw and cooked vegetables, fruits, and whole grains (brown rice, whole grain pasta, whole wheat and other whole grain breads) is most often sufficient to reestablish proper intestinal functioning.

Drinking enough water over the course of the day also encourages the intestinal transit, because the stools require a certain amount of moistness to be easily eliminated. The stools of people suffering from constipation are always dry and hard.

If necessary, one can increase the volume of roughage by adding wheat bran to the diet (1 to 3 tablespoons a day) or flaxseeds (1 to 2 tablespoons a day). These can be added to foods like yogurt and soup, for example. Both of these products have the property of swelling on contact with water, and thereby filling up the intestine.

The laxative effect of plants varies, and can thereby be easily adapted to different intestinal capacities. Chemical laxatives, however, tend to be harsh and difficult to regulate, and are to be avoided.

Gentle Laxatives

- Steep three to six prunes, or two or three dried figs in a glass of water for an entire day. That evening, eat the fruits and drink the juice.

Average Strength Laxatives

- Buckthorn in a mother tincture: take 20–70 drops with water before going to bed. You will feel the effect in the morning, upon awakening.

- Common mallow (*Malva sylvestris*) in mother tincture: take 20–50 drops with water three times a day before meals.

Strong Laxatives or Purgatives

- Castor Oil: take 1–3 capsules depending on the brand, with water in the evening.

Intestinal enemas are also extremely effective. A wide variety of these treatments exist from the rectal douche to complete cleansing of the colon via colonic irrigation. With the exception of the latter, all are easily performed in the comfort of one's home with the help of minimal equipment. Here is one example:

The Two-Quart Enema

An enema consists of the introduction of water into the colon so that the fecal matter will dissolve in the support liquid and be eliminated easily when the liquid is expelled. To introduce the water, you will need an enema bag, which can be easily purchased in most drugstores or stores specializing in health products. The enema bag also includes:

- a 2-quart container for the liquid
- a long rubber tube
- a cannula (tube suitable for insertion into the anus) with a faucet

Bring 2 quarts of water to a boil, and steep five chamomile sachets or twelve chamomile flowers for 10 minutes. Allow this to cool until it has reached a temperature of 95–98.6°F (35–37°C). Pour the "tea" through a strainer and fill the 2-quart container, placing it at a convenient height so that the water pressure will facilitate its entry into the intestines.

The part of the cannula that can be introduced into the anus should be pushed in entirely, making sure that its faucet is closed. Get down on all fours leaning your head and torso forward. Open the faucet of the cannula and allow the water to enter the intestines. It is easy to facilitate the irrigation of the intestines either by changing how deeply you are breathing, subtly shifting your position, or even by massaging your abdomen in the area directly over the colon.

If the water pressure is too strong or causes pain, close the faucet for a minute or two. Once the water has been introduced into the colon, the cannula is removed. The liquid can be held inside for several minutes to ensure that the stools are thoroughly liquefied. Then seat yourself on the toilet so that the intestinal contents can be evacuated, a process that usually takes several waves to complete.

Two-quart enemas can be performed on a daily basis for one week, or twice a week for two months. They also can be performed every now and then, as necessary.

Drainage through the Kidneys

The kidneys eliminate the wastes they filter out of the bloodstream into a back-up liquid: urine. Insufficient consumption of fluids will lead to the stagnation of toxins at the level of the filter, because they lack the support they need to take them out of the body. It is therefore important to drink enough fluids, at least half a gallon (2 liters) daily, and to eat juicy fruits and vegetables.

Medicinal plants that stimulate the kidneys to work are called diuretics. When proper doses are utilized, the volume of urine will be clearly higher than normal, or even doubled. The urine will also contain a greater amount of wastes, and consequently will assume a deeper color and thicker consistency.

The kidneys can be gently stimulated with:

- Artichoke (*Cynara cardunculus*): 1–3 tablets or capsules three times a day with water before meals.
- Pilosella (*Pilosella officinarum*) in mother tincture: three times a day, 30–50 drops with water before meals.
- Juniper Berries (*Juniperus communis*): 1 teaspoon of berries per cup, steep for 10 minutes, three cups a day.

There are also quite a few herb teas that advertise their use for "kidneys and bladder," or their "diuretic" or "renal" properties.

Drainage through the Skin

The skin expels many wastes from the body through perspiration, evidence for which is the strong body odor of people suffering ill health. Repeated periods of heavy sweating are necessary to cleanse the biological terrain thoroughly.

For those who are capable, sustained physical exercise represents the best option for perspiration, because sweat is much more concentrated when created by exertion. To encourage the process, the individual must engage in the exercise of choice (jogging, bike riding, and so on) while wearing enough clothes to accumulate the heat necessary to trigger sweating. To further assist breaking a sweat, the effort should be rather long in duration and induce sufficient exertion. At least one session a week is necessary to guarantee sufficient elimination.

The practice of taking a sauna has a long history. The only necessary precaution is that the number of sessions and the temperature of the cool bath that follows should be adapted to the vitality of the individual. Like physical exercise that induces sweating, the sauna remains a fairly athletic practice.

The High-Temperature Bath

In contrast to saunas, high-temperature baths are one of the simplest and most effective means of inducing heavy sweating. They also offer the advantage of being easy to practice at home. The patient enters a pleasant temperature bath, then gradually adds hot water until it becomes quite hot. The addition of hot water should stop just before it becomes too hot for comfort. This sensation of "too hot" varies widely from one person to the next. However, the important thing is not the objective temperature but the subjective sensation, because this is what will trigger perspiration. The individual should be able to stay in the hot bath for ten to twenty minutes.

Drinking an infusion of elder or linden flowers before the bath will facilitate perspiration (1 tablespoon per cup, let steep 10 minutes).

In addition to the heavy sweating this process triggers, another advantage of this kind of bath is the bracing effect it has on the bloodstream. In increasing circulation, it dislodges a large amount of waste from the deep tissues. To avoid an abrupt and massive exodus of these toxins toward the excretory organs, it's best to start with one weekly bath, and gradually work up to a rate of three baths a week. Several baths are sometimes necessary before the skin "opens" and sweating takes place properly.

The bath is followed by resting horizontally for at least half an hour with the body wrapped in towels or sheets. Sweating can continue during this resting period.

Drainage through the Lungs

The lungs are equipped to expel primarily gaseous wastes. However, when the biological terrain is greatly overloaded with wastes and the excretory organs are exhausted, the respiratory tract serves as a kind of emergency exit. The patient begins expectorating, spitting, and coughing up solid waste in the form of phlegm, or colloidal waste. This defensive reaction can be intentionally triggered for therapeutic purposes. In fact, all physical activity causes some degree of shortness of breath, and a more intense rate of oxygen exchange in the lungs facilitates the elimination of colloidal waste burdening the bronchia. To create this eliminatory shortness of breath, simply take a walk, jog, go for a bike ride, or walk up the stairs.

Certain medicinal plants activate this kind of elimination and make it easier by liquefying the wastes.

- Eucalyptus (*Eucalyptus globulus*): 1–3 tablets, three times a day with water before meals.
- Thyme (*Thymus vulgaris*) in a mother tincture: three times a day, 20–40 drops with water before meals.
- Coltsfoot (*Tussilago farfara*): 1 teaspoon of flowers per cup, steep 10 minutes, three to four cups a day between meals.

Dislodging the Wastes

The opening of the excretory organs allows a large number of wastes to leave the body. However, some of these wastes have been in the tissues for so long that they are now encrusted within them. They therefore need to be dislodged and sent back to a blood vessel so they can find their way out through the most appropriate excretory organ. To accomplish this, the overall circulation of fluids in the body should be activated to increase exchanges between the blood and the cellular fluids. It is also possible to "burn off" and break down wastes where they are lodged in the tissues by increasing bodily combustions through a process called autolysis.

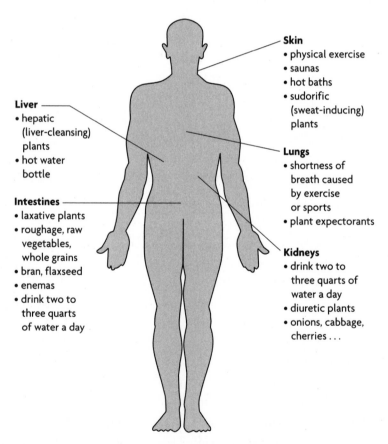

Skin
- physical exercise
- saunas
- hot baths
- sudorific (sweat-inducing) plants

Liver
- hepatic (liver-cleansing) plants
- hot water bottle

Lungs
- shortness of breath caused by exercise or sports
- plant expectorants

Intestines
- laxative plants
- roughage, raw vegetables, whole grains
- bran, flaxseed
- enemas
- drink two to three quarts of water a day

Kidneys
- drink two to three quarts of water a day
- diuretic plants
- onions, cabbage, cherries . . .

The excretory organs and their drainers

Accelerating Exchanges

The practice of a sport like bike riding, long-distance running, hiking in the mountains, and so forth vigorously stirs the bodily fluids in the depths of the tissues because of the physical exertion these exercises require. Repeated muscular contractions crush the tissues as if they were sponges, thereby setting the waste-saturated fluids of the body in motion.

Sick individuals who are no longer capable of making a sustained effort can benefit from this kind of churning of deep bodily fluids by either extremely hot baths or massage. With massage, the crushing of the tissues does not result from muscular contractions but from pressure exerted by the massage therapist. By adapting the type and strength of the massage to the individual patient, a highly beneficial acceleration of exchanges on the cellular level can be obtained.

Special mention should be made of a particular massage technique known as lymphatic drainage, which is intended to drain the lymphatic system. During this process, lymph, which normally travels quite slowly through the body, is pushed forward through the lymphatic vessels. The nodes are also encouraged to disgorge stagnating lymph in this way. The drainage of toxins and the resulting cleansing of the biological terrain through this process can often be quite remarkable.

Increasing Combustion

By increasing combustion within the body, wastes can be "burned away" on site, which offers certain advantages. All the body then has to do is eliminate the "ashes," wastes that are much tinier and easier to transport. In fact, without such a process, wastes are often too large in size to be extracted from the tissues and guided out of the body through the excretory system.

This process, in which wastes are broken down into smaller particles and digested by the body, is known as autolysis. It is caused by the activity of enzymes produced by the cells themselves, in response to special diets and fasts.

Autolysis is only triggered during particular situations when the body is not receiving sufficient nourishment. This means the body will digest its own tissues to make available to the vital organs the essential nutrients they require to function. The body withdraws nutrients from its less vital regions—for example, fat cells or muscles—to transfer them to more vital areas such as the heart, brain, or liver.

By virtue of the wisdom that governs the phenomenon of autolysis, the tissues are attacked in the reverse order of their importance, starting with those that are least important to the body's ability to function. Wastes and toxins will therefore be broken down before the more important tissues.

It is possible to trigger this autolysis of wastes and sick tissues (tumors) intentionally by following a restrictive diet. The greater the restriction of this diet, the more intense the autolysis will be.

There are a great many restrictive diets. The main thing is to reduce the quantity of different foods ingested, while keeping in mind that this is meant to be a therapeutic procedure and, as such, should be followed for only a limited time and adapted to the capacity of the patient (from several days to a week as a single cure, or repeated several times over a longer period). For cures of extended duration, it is crucial to seek the guidance of a competent health care practitioner.

When this restriction eliminates all food except water, it is a fast. If all foods but one are eliminated, it is a mono diet (grape diet, carrot diet, or similar).* Diets in which two or more foods are retained are included under the term *restrictive*. Examples include the low-calorie diet, or diets that set a limit to the number of carbohydrates or fat grams consumed during the course of a day. The restriction can be centered on one food (meat, salt) or a group of foods (red meat, fats, refined sugar). Fasts, mono diets, or restrictive diets that are adapted to the specific health needs of the individual patient figure among the most effective and useful natural means for treating disease.

A restrictive diet that is followed for a fairly extended period of time, or repeated, quite often leads to the breaking down and elimination of substantial quantities of waste. The internal biological terrain of the body, the cradle for all disease, will thereby find itself purified with a resulting improvement in overall health.

Summary: Different Kinds of Diets

- Restrictive diet: partial or complete elimination of one or several foods, as opposed to the standard diet
- Mono diet: one food plus water
- Fast: water only

⚶

Increasing combustion and accelerating the metabolism through physical exercise or high heat baths, or by triggering the process of autolysis, replicates the purifying and healing process that nature itself triggers with fever. Fever is one of the most potent healing methods employed by the

---

*For more detailed information on diets, see my book *The Detox Mono Diet: The Miracle Grape Cure and Other Cleansing Diets*, Rochester, Vt.: Healing Arts Press, 2006.

vital force of the body, and for this reason it is present in many illnesses. Fever certainly signals that the body is in danger, but it also indicates that it is still capable of fighting back. Thanks to fever, the body can compensate to a certain extent for its past shortfalls and sluggish activity by functioning more vigorously and burning away toxins that have collected in the tissues.

Some individuals suffering from ill health no longer have the physical strength necessary to "create" a fever. The methods for raising body heat described in this section on dislodging wastes are copied from nature and enable us to re-create nature's beneficial defense system.

> ✤
>
> When organs are congested, blood is dirty, the tissues poisoned, and the cells asphyxiated, there is only one logical action to be taken to restore the body to health: clean it.

BENEFITS OF EXERCISE

The benefits of physical activity are so numerous that by themselves they can compensate for, and partially eliminate, the harmful effects caused by the congestion of the biological terrain with toxins.

Increasing physical activity makes it possible to burn off the excesses created by overeating. Physical exertion activates physical functions and thereby encourages the abundant elimination of toxins. Through the acceleration of cellular exchanges and blood flow, the wastes embedded in the depths of the tissues can be dislodged and carried away to the excretory organs to be expelled from the body. The deeper breathing caused by physical exertion causes a considerable increase in the body's supply of oxygen, which encourages the breaking down of toxins and, thereby, the purification of the biological terrain.

Nothing is more capable of bringing about deep changes in the body's internal cellular environment than physical exercise. Just as a fresh breeze rekindles the almost-extinguished sparks beneath a bed of ash, exercise will reignite and cleanse the body.

But doing "physical exercise" does not refer only to those privileged and limited moments during which we visit the gym, bike, or play tennis. We also can be very physically active in our regular everyday lives if, instead of hopping into the car to drive to the office, we get there at least partially on foot; skip the elevator and take the stairs; carry our own bags; and instead of using an electric mixer or blender, beat or pulverize our foods by hand. As an added bonus, physical exercise releases endorphins, which are known to improve mental attitude.

₭

By adding only physical exercise, we can create profound changes in our biological terrain.

FILLING THE DEFICIENCIES

A sick body, if it is overloaded with wastes, is also generally suffering from deficiencies in a number of nutritive substances: vitamins, minerals, trace elements, and so on. Supplying it with these missing substances will allow it to repair its injured and depleted tissues, strengthen its organs, and resume normal functioning.

The sicker the body, the more ravenous it is for the nutrients it is lacking. Supplies of these missing nutrients need to be provided regularly and over an extended period of time. In this way, the deficiencies will be gradually satisfied and the patient's body will recover its former strength and vitality.

A healthy, natural, and varied diet would be the best way to fill the deficiencies and supply missing nutrients, if the foods available were not so often lacking in these same nutrients. For this reason, it is essential to also include nutrient-rich dietary supplements in the patient's daily intake, in order to compensate for these deficiencies as rapidly as possible.

> ℘
>
> The sicker the body, the hungrier it is for the nutrients it lacks.

A Non-Deficient Diet

The ideal non-deficient diet is the one offered by food farmed organically or biodynamically, as both of these methods respect the natural development of plants and provide the most favorable growing conditions. These farming methods produce grains, fruits, and vegetables capable of maintaining the health of those who consume them.

In order to enjoy the benefits offered by non-deficient foods, it is obviously necessary to avoid creating shortages in the food by overcooking it, for example. Additionally, all refined foods should be avoided, as some of their essential nutrients have been removed. Instead of white bread and pasta, people should eat whole grain or brown bread and whole grain pasta. Refined oils should be replaced by cold-pressed, virgin vegetable oils (except in cooking). Refined sugars should be replaced by unrefined cane sugar or other natural sweeteners like honey, maple syrup, pear concentrate, or agave. Candies and other sweets should be replaced by fresh or dried fruits.

SUGGESTED REPLACEMENTS FOR
COMMONLY EATEN FOODS

Commonly Eaten Food	Suggested Replacement
Fruits and vegetables grown by industrial farming	Fruits and vegetables grown using organic or biodynamic farming methods
White flour	Whole grain flour
White bread	Dark bread, whole grain and semi–whole grain bread
White flour pasta	Pasta made from whole grain flour
White rice	Brown rice
Refined white or brown sugar	Unrefined cane sugar, honey, maple syrup, date extract, pear concentrate, agave
Jam	Honey, whole fruit concentrate, maple cream, hazelnut or almond butter
Candy, chocolate	fresh and dried fruit, fruit butter, yogurt or kefir with fruit, fruit leather, whole grain cereal and fruit bars
White flour crackers	Whole grain crackers
Iodized kitchen salt	Sea salt, aromatic herb blends, soy sauce, gomasio (ground sesame seeds and sea salt)
Refined oil (in salad dressing)	Virgin, cold-pressed oil (sunflower, corn, olive, rapeseed, thistle, safflower)

SUGGESTED REPLACEMENTS FOR
COMMONLY EATEN FOODS (CONTINUED)

Commonly Eaten Food	Suggested Replacement
Coffee	Roasted grain beverage coffee substitute
Black tea	Herb tea
Commercial carbonated beverages	Mineral water, herb tea, fruit or vegetable juice, juice mixed with seltzer water

By eating a variety of foods, one will avoid a unilateral diet, which is one of the main causes of nutritive deficiencies. In short, to avoid scarcities in your diet and the deficiencies that then appear in your body, eat a varied diet composed of whole grain and organically grown foods.

Food Supplements

The healing process can be accelerated, thanks to the use of pollen (bee and flower), brewer's yeast, various seaweed products, cod liver oil, spirulina, blackstrap molasses, wheat germ, royal jelly, and so on. The strong concentrations of vitamins and minerals contained in these foods, and their easy assimilation by the body, helps fill deficiencies much more rapidly because of the quantity, quality, and variety of nutrients they supply. In fact, each nutrient depends to some extent on the presence of other nutrients in order to be assimilated properly.

Since certain food supplements are more effective for some patients than others, it's important to look for advice, or experiment to find the most suitable options. Healing by means of these supplements can take several weeks, or even months.

It is possible to take several different products at the same time without any adverse effects.

SOME OF THE CRUCIAL FOOD SUPPLEMENTS

Vitamin supplements	Bee pollen, brewer's yeast (in powder or liquid), sprouted grains, wheat germ and flaxseed oil, concentrates of acerola or sea buckthorn, spirulina
Minerals and trace elements	Tablets made from powdered bone, seaweed, or shell; sea water (Quinton products); magnesium; blackstrap molasses; spring water; horsetail
General revitalizers	Royal jelly, ginseng, fish roe, a cocktail made from liquid yeast and fruit and vegetable juice

> ❧
>
> By repairing deficiencies, the sick individual is better able to eliminate toxins; likewise, when the body rids itself of toxins, it's easier to supplement deficiencies. The two processes are inseparably bound together.

RESTORING THE ACID-ALKALINE BALANCE

An overacidic biological terrain is corrected primarily by means of food. Rather than consuming more acidifying foods than alkaline foods, as is generally the case, the individual must keep track of what is eaten to see that the proportion is equal, or even reduce the proportion of acidic foods to fall below that of alkaline foods. The proportion of alkalizing foods consumed should be 50 percent in an individual with a normal pH balance, but 60 to 80 percent in someone with overacidity. Simply put, this means eating more vegetables—green salads, raw and cooked vegetables, potatoes—than meat and flour products. An additional measure aims at eliminating all foods containing refined white sugar, which is, in fact, a powerful acidifying agent.

Alkaline foods that must be increased to make up for the acidifying foods are all the green and colorful vegetables, which come in great variety. Potatoes, which are extremely alkalizing, should replace grains as often as possible, although grains should not be totally excluded from the diet. Chestnuts, almonds, avocadoes, dates, and bananas are other foods that are highly alkalizing. Dairy products such as cottage cheese along with eggs are balanced proteins to substitute for meat and fish. Whole sugar from the cane or agave nectar should be used in the place of white sugar, and maple syrup, fruit concentrate, and honey can take the place of preserves and jellies.

Acidifying Foods

These foods may seem to be alkaline in nature, but make the body's pH more acidic:

- Red meat, fowl, processed meat products, meat extracts, fish, shellfish (mussels, shrimp, and so on)
- Eggs
- Cheese (strong cheese is more acidic than mild cheese)
- Animal fat (lard, suet)

- Vegetable oil, especially peanut and refined oil, and oil spreads (margarine)
- Whole and refined grains: wheat, oats, and especially millet
- Bread, pasta, cereal flakes, and all foods made from refined grains
- Legumes: peanuts and beans (soy, white, broad, navy, and so on)
- White sugar
- Sweets: syrup, pastry, chocolate, candy, preserves, jellied fruits
- Oleaginous fruits: walnuts, hazelnuts, pumpkin seeds, and so on (except chestnuts and almonds)
- Commercially made sodas, sodas with cola base and others
- Coffee, tea, cocoa, wine
- Condiments such as mayonnaise, mustard, and ketchup

Alkalizing Foods

These foods help to combat overacidity and restore acid-alkaline balance:

- Potatoes
- Green vegetables of all types (raw or cooked), salad greens
- Colorful vegetables: carrots, beets, red and yellow peppers, and so on (except tomatoes)
- Corn (kernels or cooked as polenta)
- Milk (liquid or powder), cream, butter, well-drained cottage cheese
- Bananas
- Almonds, Brazil nuts

- Chestnuts
- Dried fruits, especially dates and raisins (except those that are tart to the taste: apricots, apples, and so on)
- Alkaline mineral water
- Almond milk
- Black olives preserved in oil
- Avocadoes
- Cold-pressed oil
- Natural sugar

Weak Acid Foods

The acidifying effects of these foods vary according to the individual's ability to metabolize acids:

- Whey, yogurt, curdled milk, kefir, cottage cheese that has not been drained well
- Fresh fruits (the less ripe the fruit, the greater the acidity)
- Fruit juice
- Sauerkraut, lacto-fermented vegetables
- Honey
- Vinegar

Setting aside the dietary factor, there are other measures that should be taken. Better oxidation of acids occurs when there is physical activity—such as walking, sports, gardening—and elimination of acids already present in the tissues can be increased by the consumption of diuretic medicinal plants (for the kidneys) and sudorifics, or sweat-inducing plants, for the skin.

Another extremely important measure, one proven essential for most cases, is the taking of alkaline mineral supplements to help the body not only eliminate acids ingested daily, but also, and primarily, to facilitate the evacuation of acids lodged in the depths of the tissues. This measure is of major importance because the body resists allowing acids embedded in the tissues to be pulled back into the bloodstream—en route to the excretory organs—because their return to the bloodstream represents a dangerous alteration of its pH. These acids, therefore, have an unfortunate tendency to be kept in the depths of the tissues to protect the blood. However, a substantial delivery of alkaline reserves to the body makes it possible to eliminate these embedded acids. Buffered by the alkaline supplements, the acids can drift back to the surface in the form of neutral salts, a form that will not harm the blood pH.

Alkaline supplements are blends of calcium, magnesium, potassium, and so forth in a form easily assimilated by the body. Available in tablet form or powder, these preparations are to be taken three times a day with a little water, before meals. To assure appropriate dosage, it should be calibrated in accordance with the urinary pH of the individual concerned. The general rule is to take as much supplement as necessary to obtain a urinary pH between 7 and 7.5, based on the second and subsequent urinations of the day (not the first one). Therefore, if a dose of 2 tablets, three times a day pushes the pH from 5.5 to 6.5, the dosage will have to be increased so that it can get to a normal pH of 7 to 7.5. This important rule ensures that correction of the acidity in the biological terrain is done properly.

The various measures undertaken to deacidify the biological terrain will gradually cause all the acids embedded in the depth of the tissues to come to the surface and be expelled from the body. Over time, this deacidification of the depths of the biological terrain will not only heal the patient from current ills, but also prevent any relapses.

SPECIFIC REMEDIES

In addition to the general therapeutic maneuvers described in this chapter, it is sometimes necessary to give additional support to the weak points of the body. Treatment ceases to be general, focused on the entire biological terrain, but addresses a specific organ, strengthens a deficient function, soothes irritable tissues, disinfects, and so on. Every patient has vulnerable points that need to be taken into consideration during treatment, along with the major steps being taken to correct the biological terrain.

Among specific remedies that can be utilized are such dissimilar but effective therapies as medicinal plants, aromatherapy, magnetics, homeopathy, facial and foot reflexology, acupuncture, hydrotherapy, and many more. But, let me repeat, these specific treatments should all be employed as complements to the overall treatment of the biological terrain.

POSITIVE MENTAL ATTITUDE

The tool we know as the human body functions in accordance with its own inner logic, but it is also highly influenced by our mental life. A balanced nature, confronting life with confidence, trust, and optimism provides the most favorable conditions for the body's harmonious functioning. Conversely, negativity, fear, and aggressive attitudes disrupt this functioning and slow it down, and can throw the body completely off kilter. The physical state espouses the fluctuations of thoughts and emotions. Physical functioning so clearly mirrors state of mind that it is often enough for a patient to believe his illness is growing worse for it actually to become worse.

Depending on the patient's mental attitude, the healing process can be hampered and blocked, or, to the contrary, supported and even stimulated. It is therefore of enormous consequence that the patient adopt an appropriate attitude in confronting his illness. How can the body keep fighting if the patient has abandoned the struggle, or even worse, is fighting the healing process? The will to get better, along with active participation in the remedial treatment by freeing the body from the pressure of negative thoughts, mobilizes the defense system and supports regeneration.

Conclusion

ॐ

A clear and realistic vision regards the human body as a tool that has been placed at our disposal. This tool functions in accordance with precise instructions that must be followed to maintain its proper working order. In other words, there are a certain number of physiological imperatives—laws of health—that set out conditions for the proper functioning of the body. The body must be used and maintained in conformance with these instructions, and not as momentary moods, whims, and desires dictate. A person loses healthy equilibrium and falls ill when the laws of health, as described in this book, are not respected. As long as they are adhered to, the body will remain in excellent health.

Every disease has a cause. Its very existence necessarily implies mistakes have been made in the physical and mental circumstances of the person afflicted. So long as these errors are not detected and eliminated, health problems will persist and be provoked. It is therefore absolutely necessary to alter one's personal health regimen. *Changes* must take place. The patient can and should take control by beginning to eat differently, eliminating the sources of toxic buildup, leading a more physically active life, or adopting a new mental attitude.

Therapeutic methods are available to help the patient, but these changes are something that only the patient, not the naturopath, can make happen. If the naturopath leans toward optimism, it is not for the purpose of planting suggestions that will encourage healing in the patient's mind. The confidence and hope the naturopath can give is based on a concrete reality, one confirmed by countless cases of remission and healing.

Now, in closing, I leave you with a summary of six basic rules for recovering and maintaining health:

1. Eat a varied diet of whole, preferably organic foods, consisting predominantly of plants.

2. Eat too little rather than too much.

3. Drink more than 2 quarts of water a day.

4. Engage in physical activity every day.

5. Get enough sleep every night.

6. Approach all of life's challenges with a positive and constructive attitude.

Glossary of the Concepts
of Naturopathy

ॐ

The numbers following each definition refer the reader to
pages in the book where the concept is discussed.

acid-alkaline balance: This is the balance between acid and
alkaline substances in the body that permits it to remain in
good health. The unit used to measure the degree of acidity
or alkalinity is pH (*see also* pH). The normal pH of blood,
and of the biological terrain in general, is 7.39. When there is
movement away from this ideal pH, disease appears. Acidosis, or excess acid, is the most common example of an acid-
alkaline imbalance, and is a common result of our acidifying
lifestyle and diet. Acidosis can be corrected by following an
alkalizing diet, oxygenation, and by taking alkaline supplements. (67, 101)

acidosis: The state of the body when the acid-alkaline ratio is
out of balance and the biological terrain is acidic. (68)

acute and chronic illness: Diseases are crises of detoxification
or cleansing triggered by the vital force as it seeks to eliminate
the surplus of toxins encumbering the biological terrain. An
illness is acute when the vital force is strong. Elimination is
violent, spectacular, and short in duration . . . and it achieves

its goal: the renewal of the biological terrain. Chronic diseases are the same efforts made by a weakened vital force, and are, therefore, of lesser intensity. Incapable of repairing the biological terrain in one attempt, these crises will recur regularly, hence their chronic nature. (30)

allopathic medicine: A therapeutic method that deals with disease by using methods that, generally speaking, oppose the curative effects of the body's vital force. By repressing toxins into the depths of the body, anti-symptom remedies are successful in banishing symptoms from the surface, but this is to the detriment of the biological terrain. The opposite method of health care is naturopathy. (3)

autolysis: Autolysis is a physiological process triggered by special diets and fasts during which the body digests or breaks down (*lyse*) its own tissues (*auto*). When it stops receiving any or enough nutrients from outside, the body is forced to draw on its own reserves for nutritive substances, which it does by first self-digesting diseased tissue and toxins. Autolysis, therefore, has a curative effect because it rids the biological terrain of the wastes with which it is encumbered. (94)

biological terrain: Just as a plant will either prosper or wither depending on the quality of the terrain in which it grows, our cells and the organs they form will function properly or not depending on the "biological terrain" in which they find themselves. This biological terrain is composed of the bodily fluids in which the cells are immersed, in other words the fluids around them (extracellular fluid, lymph, and blood) and those inside them (intracellular fluid).

The liquid environment of the cell ensures it receives the supplies of oxygen and nutrients it needs, and thereby, this environment is the ultimate guarantor of health. Because of its crucial function, any overly large quantitative or qualitative alteration suffered by these fluids leads to disease. Two primary imbalances are possible: either the presence of an excessive amount of certain substances (toxins, poisons), which leads to diseases caused by overloads; or the absence of certain substances (nutrients, minerals), which will engender deficiency-caused diseases. (3)

chronic illness: *See* Acute and chronic illness.

colloidal waste: Colloidal waste is one of the primary varieties of toxins (*see also* Crystals). These toxins are non-soluble in liquids. For example, phlegm, the viscous substance that is eliminated by blowing one's nose, is a colloidal waste. When mixed with water these substances do not dissolve, but retain their appearance. Sputum, pus, and so on are all colloidal wastes.

Colloidal wastes are eliminated by the liver, the intestines, the sebaceous glands, and also sometimes by the lungs. The illnesses caused by colloidal wastes are not painful as those caused by crystals are, and they are fluid in nature: inflammations of the respiratory tract, acne, oozing eczema, and so forth.

The sources of colloidal waste are starches and fats. (10)

crises—cleansing, healing, detoxification: The vital force governing the body does not remain a passive bystander when confronted by the collection of toxins in the biological terrain. When the tolerance threshold has been crossed, it abruptly intensifies the functioning of one or more excretory organs to rid itself of the wastes with which it is encumbered, giving rise to the description of a cleansing, or detoxification crisis. These crises are also curative, because by eliminating the primary cause of illness—the accumulation of toxins in the biological terrain—they banish the health problem. (15)

crystals: Crystals are one of the two major kinds of waste (*see also* Colloidal waste). They are hard and can wound like real crystals, but like sugar or salt, they dissolve in water. Crystals are eliminated by the excretory organs that evacuate liquids—the kidneys and the sweat glands.

Crystals are generally acidic, like uric acid or oxalic acid, but also can be discarded mineral salts. The sand we have in our eyes when waking, and the substance that makes our joints creak are composed of crystals. Crystalloid diseases such as rheumatism, kidney stones, sciatica, tendinitis, dry eczema, and neuritis can be painful and are not "runny."

The sources of crystals are proteins, white sugar, and acidifying foods. (10)

deficiencies: A deficiency is the absence or insufficient amount of an element that is essential for the body's nutrition. The shortage may be of protein, calcium, vitamins, or any other nutritive substance. Deficiencies can involve one or more nutrients, and be temporary or long-lasting. They also can be major or minor depending on the importance of the missing substance. In deficiencies of supply, the missing nutrient does not reach the body because the food containing it is not eaten or has been extracted from the food before consumption; the refining process, for example, strips grains of their vitamin B content. In deficiencies of utilization, nutrients enter the body via their host foods, but are destroyed by harmful substances (anti-vitamins or chelators—drugs or other substances that inhibit the metabolic action of a vitamin or trace element) before the body can use them. Deficiency-based diseases are treated by providing the missing substance in order to satisfy the deficiency. (11)

depurative: A drainer that works on several excretory organs. (84)

diagnosis: In allopathic medicine, a diagnosis is made to determine what illness is afflicting the patient. The goal of a diagnosis is to identify a malady before prescribing a specific remedy. In naturopathy, there is a diagnosis but it evaluates the overall health of the individual (*see also* Health assessment). (22)

diet: Diet is one of the primary factors for remaining in, or restoring, good health. The body is entirely dependent on food for building and repairing itself, and for carrying out its functions. A poor diet causes the deficiencies and toxins that are at the root of any degradation of the biological terrain. (9, 76, 98)

dietary supplement: A product taken to supplement one's regular diet because of its richness in nutrients. Vitamins, minerals, trace elements, flower and bee pollen, brewer's yeast, seaweed and kelp, wheat germ, and spirulina are some of the many dietary supplements available. (100)

disassimilation: The passage of toxins through the intestinal mucous membranes (600 square meters or 1968 square feet of surface). The intestines, like all the excretory organs, filter the blood that passes through their tissues to remove the wastes. These wastes are then eliminated with fecal matter. (85)

diuretics: Medicinal plants that stimulate the kidneys to work. When proper doses are utilized, the volume of urine will increase and possibly double. The urine will also contain a greater amount of wastes; consequently, it will assume a deeper color and thicker consistency. (88)

drainers: Products that encourage the drainage of toxins from the body by stimulating the function of the excretory organs. These are medicinal plants or other products that have hepatic, laxative, diuretic, or similar properties. (20, 83, 93)

drainage: Drainage is a process that intentionally triggers the elimination of toxins from the body. The purpose is to reestablish normal elimination if it has been insufficient, and even to increase it for a while in order to compensate for the previous period of insufficiency.

The excretory organs are the essential vehicles for drainage. During this period, the work performed by the liver, intestines, kidneys, skin, and lungs is stimulated through a variety of techniques and cleanses. These can include medicinal plants, juice or food that has detoxifying properties, inducement of heavy sweating, poultices, intestinal enemas, and the like.

Depending on the strength of the individual patient, a drainage can be performed through one or several excretory organs. (19)

elimination: Evacuation through the excretory organs (liver, kidneys, and so on) of toxins burdening the biological terrain and becoming the source of disease. The elimination of toxins is encouraged by diet, exercise, and drainage. Health is regained through correction of the biological terrain. (18)

excretory organs: The excretory organs, or emunctories, are responsible for filtering all the metabolic residue and waste out of the blood so it can be expelled from the body. They are, therefore, not only "doors" that can be opened to allow the passage of toxins, but organs that actively cleanse the blood for the purpose of purifying it.

These organs include the liver (evacuates waste in bile), intestines (stool), kidneys (urine), lungs (exhalation), sweat glands (perspiration), and the sebaceous glands (sebum).

When they are functioning properly, the excretory organs eliminate all the wastes that are ingested or produced by a normal lifestyle. Their capacities can be exceeded by an excess production of wastes, which happens, for example, when a sedentary lifestyle is combined with overeating: toxins are not evacuated, the biological terrain deteriorates, and disease appears. (6, 19)

extracellular fluid: *See* Intracellular and extracellular fluids.

fast: A period of time during which a person abstains from any nutritional intake other than water. No food of any kind is consumed. This regimen aims at forcing the body to survive through breaking down and digesting toxins and sick tissues (autolysis), which eliminates them from the biological terrain and brings about a return to health. (21, 94)

fever: Fever is not a disease per se but a reflection of the body's attempt to defend itself from a biological terrain overloaded with toxins. Depending on the individual case, it may occur in tandem with a bacterial infection. The acceleration of immune defenses, blood circulation, respiration, and cellular exchanges produces heat and thereby increases body temperature. Fever is, therefore, a manifestation of the body defending itself, which is why it is a common symptom of so many different maladies.

If fever did not occur naturally it would need to be devised; it is a brilliant way of enabling the body to incinerate and eliminate a large amount of toxins in a short space of time. Unless the patient's temperature climbs so high that it poses risks to the body, breaking a fever amounts to obstructing the body's defense system. (31)

filling the deficiencies: This is the action of supplying missing nutrients to the body to alleviate deficiencies. In this expression, deficiencies are viewed as holes to be plugged by filling them with the missing nutrients. (98)

healing: Healing represents the return to health after an illness. A true healing takes place when the symptoms of the disease, as well as the deficiencies of the biological terrain that engendered them, have vanished. This new state of health is stable and lasting because the primary causes of the disease have been eliminated.

Healings obtained locally by treatments targeting only the symptoms are fictitious, as these treatments are satisfied with burying the toxins in the depths of the body without correcting the biological terrain. Although seeming to be cured, the patient's biological terrain remains in a degraded state. (23)

health: Health is not the absence of detectable disease symptoms, but corresponds to a state of the biological terrain in which the composition of the bodily fluids ensures and provides the conditions favorable to the cells' unhampered normal activity. Health is determined by the state of the body's internal cellular environment. If this biological terrain is healthy, then the body is healthy; if it is unhealthy, the body is ill, even if there are no apparent symptoms.

Because the biological terrain is dependent on our health and lifestyle decisions, health is an unstable equilibrium that is constantly menaced by overloads and deficiencies. The balance represented by good health is not acquired once and for all, but requires constant vigilance to maintain. (5)

health assessment: An analysis of the patient's diet, eliminatory capacity, and self-care to determine what has degraded the biological terrain and caused the manifestation of specific localized disorders. The health assessment does not determine which anti-symptom remedies are required, but suggests measures for draining toxins out of the body, filling its deficiencies, giving support to under-performing organs, and reforming the patient's self-care and awareness as necessary. These measures correct the biological terrain, thereby bringing about the elimination of the symptoms of disease. (23)

hepatic: A person suffering from liver ailments. Also, a product or substance that stimulates the elimination of waste by the liver. Through the taking of hepatic plants (dandelion, boldo, rosemary), the liver filters more waste out of the bloodstream, which leads to an increased production of bile. A hepatic reaction can also be obtained with a hot water bottle. (70, 84)

hygiene: All the methods (diet, exercise, rest, and so on) taken together that can be implemented for restoring or preserving health. A method based on hygiene seeks to adapt the lifestyle to the body's capacity, whereas an anti-symptom therapy too often consists only of adapting the physical capacities to the lifestyle. (11)

iatrogenic: This designates a health problem resulting from the medication prescribed to heal the patient, sometimes described as side effects. This type of event is extremely rare in naturopathy, but much more common with the use of anti-symptom remedies in allopathic medicine. (24)

immune response: The body's ability to defend itself not only when confronted by germs, but also when faced with various toxins that clog the biological terrain. (16)

internal cellular environment: *See* Biological terrain.

intracellular and extracellular fluids: Fluids found both inside (intra) and outside (extra) the cells. This is the cellular serum, a pale white liquid. It has almost the same composition as blood, but without blood's red corpuscles.

The extracellular fluid, which represents 15 percent of the weight of the body, constitutes the external environment of the cells. This substance carries oxygen and nutrients to the cells, and carries away wastes they expel, toward the excretory organs.

Intracellular fluid represents 50 percent of the weight of the body. It fills the cells, gives the body shape and tone, and allows the exchanges that need to take place between organs. (4)

intrinsic illness: The constricted state of the body's internal cellular environment caused by toxins in the biological terrain that exceed the body's capacity for restoring its own balance. (6)

laxative: Any product or substance that stimulates the elimination of intestinal waste. A laxative effect is induced with plants such as alder buckthorn and mallow, or through enemas, abdominal massage, and so on. A laxative gently stimulates intestinal peristalsis, encouraging regular evacuation of stools. The term *purgative* is reserved for products that powerfully stimulate the intestines and bring about the rapid and complete emptying of their contents. (21, 86)

laws of health: These are the physiological imperatives to which the body is subject and from which it cannot escape, and which compel us to act in a specific manner in order to stay healthy. Eating enough raw food to cover the body's nutrient needs, for example, is one law of health, because the body inevitably will fall ill if it does not get them. Drinking enough water on a daily basis, getting sufficient physical exercise, regularly eliminating toxins produced by the body, and so on are all laws of health. (108)

metabolism: Metabolism refers to all the biochemical transformations that take place in the body tissue during digestion, assimilation, energy production, catabolism, exchanges, and so forth. Waste and residue, called toxins, are the result of these transformations and need to be eliminated through the excretory organs. (9–10)

mono diets: During the course of a mono diet, only one (mono) food is consumed. Each meal consists exclusively of the food in question, eaten either raw or cooked, or as juice when possible. The most common mono diets use grapes, carrots, or rice. (21, 94)

naturopathy: Naturopathy is a therapeutic method that treats disease using natural methods and takes action to improve the biological terrain rather than to diminish symptoms. In supporting the body's own healing power, it addresses the deep roots of illness rather than the effects, and employs a variety of natural techniques as listed below. (1, 3, 7)

Nutrition

- Healthy diet: organic foods; unrefined, whole grain foods without additives
- Restrictive and dietetic diets: fasts, mono diets, food-combining diets, natural foods diets
- Nutritional diets to make up for deficiencies
- Natural food supplements

Water Therapies

- Cold and hot hydrotherapy
- Balneotherapy, thermal and mud baths
- Enemas

Exercise

- Moderate exercise, gentle gymnastics, body building, martial arts, sports

Plant Therapies

- Medicinal plants in their various forms: infusions, decoctions, mother tinctures, essential oils
- Fruits and vegetables with healing properties

Massage

- Different types of massage: whole body, specific region, sports, deep tissue, French, Swedish, Chinese, Thai; chiropractic; osteopathy

Reflexology

- Stimulation of the reflex zones of the feet, hands, ears, nose, or back

Light Therapies

- Beneficial effects of the sun (heliotherapy), influence of the moon and stars
- Colors and their properties

Air

- Breathing techniques
- Oxygenation
- Aromatherapy

Energetic Techniques

- Therapeutic magnets
- Revitalization through the magnetism of precious and semi-precious stones and their benefits
- Earth energies

Mental Attitude

- Importance of thoughts and attitudes, mental health
- Stress management
- Relaxation, self-suggestion, visualization
- Sleep

nutrients: Substances necessary for the construction and functioning of the body that are normally provided by food. These include proteins, carbohydrates, fats, minerals, trace elements, and vitamins. (37)

opening the excretory organs: Increasing the elimination of toxins through the body's excretory organs. This is recommended when these organs are working too slowly or are "closed," or clearly functioning below normal. (83)

overloads: Wastes, toxins, and toxic by-products, including fats but not exclusively, that dangerously burden the biological terrain when they collect in overly large quantities; in other words, they overload it. This has nothing to with being overweight, but rather having an excess of all kinds of toxins. (8)

pH: Measuring unit for the degree of acidity or alkalinity of a substance; pH is shorthand for the substance's potential (p) or power to free hydrogen (H) ions. The measuring scale goes from 0 to 14: 0 is absolute acidity, 14 absolute alkalinity, and 7 is the middle position known as neutral pH. The optimal pH of the blood and the biological terrain is slightly alkaline: 7.39. (43, 67)

plurality of disease: The concept that each disease is unique by nature and has causes specific to it and dissimilar from those of other illnesses. There are, therefore, no common elements among disparate diseases. This concept in allopathic medicine leads practitioners to treat every disease with a specific remedy (therapeutic plurality).

This concept is diametrically opposed to the single cause, or unity of disease that is the foundation of naturopathy. (3)

purify: To purify is to make clean. In naturopathy, this word refers to all the efforts deployed to rid the blood and the biological terrain of toxins. (21)

relapse: When an illness, bronchitis for example, has been cleared up using only an anti-symptom treatment, the biological terrain will not have been corrected and the vital force will make renewed attempts to purify the internal cellular environment. Each of these attempts may manifest at another excretory organ (*see* transfer of disease) or on the same organ. In the latter case, the illness is referred to as a relapse. The toxins that have been pushed into the body's depths by the anti-symptom treatment find their way back to the excretory organ used initially. One case of bronchitis is soon followed by another case of bronchitis. It is sometimes believed that this is the appearance of a new case of illness, but in fact it is the same healing crisis that was momentarily interrupted, but is triggered anew as soon as circumstances permit. (26)

remedy: Product containing active substances for treating illness. In naturopathy, remedies are not used to cause the arbitrary disappearance of symptoms without taking any action on the biological terrain. To the contrary, they aim to support elimination via the excretory organs in order to correct the body's internal cellular environment, where the root of the problem is located. This correction will automatically bring about the disappearance of the symptoms. (14)

restrictive diet: A diet characterized by a reduced quantity of foods (low calorie, low salt, and so forth) or by a reduction in the scope of foods permitted (meatless, salt-free, fat-free, and so on). Such diets aim to bring relief to the body and trigger the process of autolysis to eliminate toxins. (94)

sedentary lifestyle: A state in which the motor capacities of the body are underutilized either because of a job that requires the worker to remain seated, the use of motor vehicles to travel rather than walk even for short distances, the absence of physical activity during leisure times, or all of the above. A sedentary lifestyle weakens the muscles and organs, causes under-oxygenation, slowed metabolism of food intake, and poor elimination of toxins. (62)

self-healing: Remedies alone are incapable of healing a patient. They can only restore, support, or reinforce the healing process implemented by the vital force that animates and guides the body. In this sense, healing does not come from the outside but from within the body. The vital force corresponds with what the ancients called the medicalizing nature, which we know as the immune response.

The body is, therefore, capable of working alone to effect its own healing, in other words, self-healing. "It is nature that heals disease, and medicine is the art of imitating the healing procedures of nature," wrote Hippocrates. Somewhat later in time, the famous French surgeon Ambroise Paré (1509–1590) would say: "I dress wounds; it is nature that heals them." (16)

self-poisoning: This kind of poisoning comes from toxins not outside, but within the body. It begins in the intestines when they are unable to empty properly or well. The poisons, toxins, and wastes that result from fermentation and putrefaction, and are not rapidly evacuated in stools, are absorbed into the intestinal walls and then enter the bloodstream. From there they are conducted all over the body, initiating self-poisoning. (38)

sudorific: Any product or substance that stimulates the elimination of toxins through the sudoriferous (sweat) glands. Saunas, hot baths, and exercise have a sweat-inducing effect, as do medicinal plants such as linden and elder flowers. All of these cause the glands to expel a greater quantity of sweat, which will have a higher content of toxins. (89, 104)

supplies: Everything taken in by the body that allows it to function—food, vitamins, water, oxygen, and so on. (4, 11)

symptoms: Symptoms are the surface manifestations of the deep-rooted illness of the deteriorated biological terrain. All the symptoms of a disease, such as the inflamed and painful joints of rheumatism, are often considered to be the intrinsic disease. In reality, the true disease is the degraded biological terrain that has allowed these symptoms to manifest. (2)

toxins: Toxins are the wastes and residues created by the metabolic process. The largest quantity of toxins comes from the breaking down of food substances by the body. For example, used proteins create urea, uric acid, and creatine; the combustion of glucose produces lactic acid; poorly transformed fats turn into ketonic acid, and so forth.

Another portion of bodily toxins is produced by wear and tear on the tissues. This includes the debris of dead cells, vestiges of red corpuscles, exhausted minerals, and so on.

Other toxins are poisons that come into the body from the outside and are not part of the normal biological cycle: heavy metals from pollution (mercury, cadmium), insecticides, herbicides, preservatives, food additives, and the list goes on. To be precise, the word *toxin* should be applied only to wastes produced by the body; however, the toxic substances described here are also commonly referred to as toxins. (4, 9)

transfer of disease: The vital force of the body constantly seeks to rid the biological terrain of excess toxins, which, in addition to normal eliminations, can be revealed by more consequential evacuations from the skin (pimples, eczema), lungs (coughing), and so on. When this effort is countered by an anti-symptom treatment, the vital force does not abandon its efforts, but may transfer the excess toxins to another excretory organ. For example, wastes present in the skin will be redirected to the lungs to be eliminated from the body. This is how eczema "turns into" a cough. (26)

unity of disease: This concept of disease, which is distinctive to natural medicine, believes all health disorders are the expression of a single illness: the degradation of the biological terrain. Diseases are, therefore, only various surface manifestations of a unique, deeply rooted health problem. Hence the fundamental naturopathic aphorism, "There are no local diseases; there are only general diseases."

As the degradation of the biological terrain is always the origin for any disease, and thereby necessarily precedes the appearance of any local health problems, therapy is always essentially the same (therapeutic uniqueness): correct this internal cellular environment by ridding it of any overloads and by filling its deficiencies.

Hippocrates, the father of medicine, said in this regard: "The nature of all illness is the same. It differs only in its seat. I think it only reveals itself in such diversity because of the multiplicity of places where the illness is established. In fact, its essence is one, and the cause producing it is also one." (7, 18)

vital force: The vital force organizes living matter and orchestrates, synchronizes, and harmonizes all its organic functions. It is intangible and therefore cannot be identified with any single organ of the body. Its existence is revealed only by its effects. All of its efforts are aimed at maintaining the body in the optimum state of health. It is this force that enlivens the organs and governs the processes of respiration, circulation, digestion, exchanges, and elimination. It also triggers the reactions of the body's defense system; it scars wounds, neutralizes poisons, and prompts healing crises.

It is an intelligent force that acts wisely for the good of the organism. Hippocrates believed the medical practitioner should be "the interpreter and minister" of this medicalizing force; in other words, the therapy should reflect and mimic this force. (14)

warning signals: Minor health problems that warn us when the biological terrain is out of balance and beginning to break down. It could be not feeling well, fatigue, nervous tension, or even a few pimples or minor digestive disorder. The overload rate is still low, but correction of the lifestyle must be quickly implemented to avoid continued deterioration of the biological terrain. (29)

waste: A combination of toxins and toxic substances that degrade the biological terrain. (5)

Bibliography

꒰ᔓ꒱

Cabot, Sandra, and Marie-France Muller. *Régénérez votre foie!* St.-Julien-en-Genevois, France: Editions Jouvence, 2004.

Carton, Paul. *The Ten Commandments of Health and Happiness.* New York: Deronda Publishing Company, 1929.

Davis, Adele. *Let's Eat Right to Keep Fit.* New York: Signet, 1970.

Lust, Benedict. *Zone Therapy: Relieving Pain and Sickness by Nerve Pressure.* Chicago: Kessinger, 2003.

Lust, Benedict, and Louis Kuhne. *Neo Naturopathy: The New Science of Healing or the Unity of Diseases.* Chicago: Kessinger, 2003.

Mignot, Josiane. *Hydrotherapie du colon.* St.-Julien-en-Genevois, France: Editions Jouvence, 2005.

Valnet, Jean. *The Practice of Aromatherapy: A Classic Compendium of Plant Medicines and Their Healing Properties.* Edited by Robert Tisserand. Rochester, Vt.: Healing Arts Press, 1982, 1990.

Vasey, Christopher. *The Acid–Alkaline Diet for Optimum Health: Restore Your Health by Creating pH Balance in Your Diet.* Rochester, Vt.: Healing Arts Press, 2002. Second edition, 2006.

———. *Les compléments alimentaires naturels.* St.-Julien-en-Genevois, France: Editions Jouvence, 2003.

———. *The Detox Mono Diet.* Rochester, Vt.: Healing Arts Press, 2006.

———. *The Water Prescription.* Rochester, Vt.: Healing Arts Press, 2006.

———. *The Whey Prescription.* Rochester, Vt.: Healing Arts Press, 2006.

Resources

To find a local naturopathic physician, visit the website of the American Association of Naturopathic Physicians: **www.naturopathic.org.**

In Canada, use the search function provided by the Canadian Association of Naturopathic Doctors: **www.cand.ca.**

ALKALINE SUPPLEMENTS

pHion Nutrition
14201 N. Hayden Road, Suite A4
Scottsdale, AZ 85260
888-744-8589
www.phionbalance.com

pHion Nutrition manufactures and distributes pH test strips, alkalizing supplements, and other products geared toward detoxifying and augmenting healthy body chemistry.

AUTHOR'S WEBSITE

www.christophervasey.ch

The author presents his different books and provides for each the table of contents and a general introduction to the subject of the book. The website also contains biographical information, a calendar of conferences, and contact information.

Index

૱

BOOKS OF RELATED INTEREST

The Acid–Alkaline Diet for Optimum Health
Restore Your Health by Creating pH Balance in Your Diet
by Christopher Vasey, N.D.

The Detox Mono Diet
The Miracle Grape Cure and Other Cleansing Diets
by Christopher Vasey, N.D.

The Whey Prescription
The Healing Miracle in Milk
by Christopher Vasey, N.D.

The Water Prescription
For Health, Vitality, and Rejuvenation
by Christopher Vasey, N.D.

Traditional Foods Are Your Best Medicine
Improving Health and Longevity with Native Nutrition
by Ronald F. Schmid, N.D.

Optimal Digestive Health: A Complete Guide
Edited by Trent W. Nichols, M.D.,
and Nancy Faass, MSW, MPH

The Seasonal Detox Diet
Remedies from the Ancient Cookfire
by Carrie L'Esperance

Food Allergies and Food Intolerance
The Complete Guide to Their Identification and Treatment
by Jonathan Brostoff, M.D., and Linda Gamlin

INNER TRADITIONS • BEAR & COMPANY
P.O. Box 388
Rochester, VT 05767
1-800-246-8648
www.InnerTraditions.com
Or contact your local bookseller